EVERYDAY WELLNESS

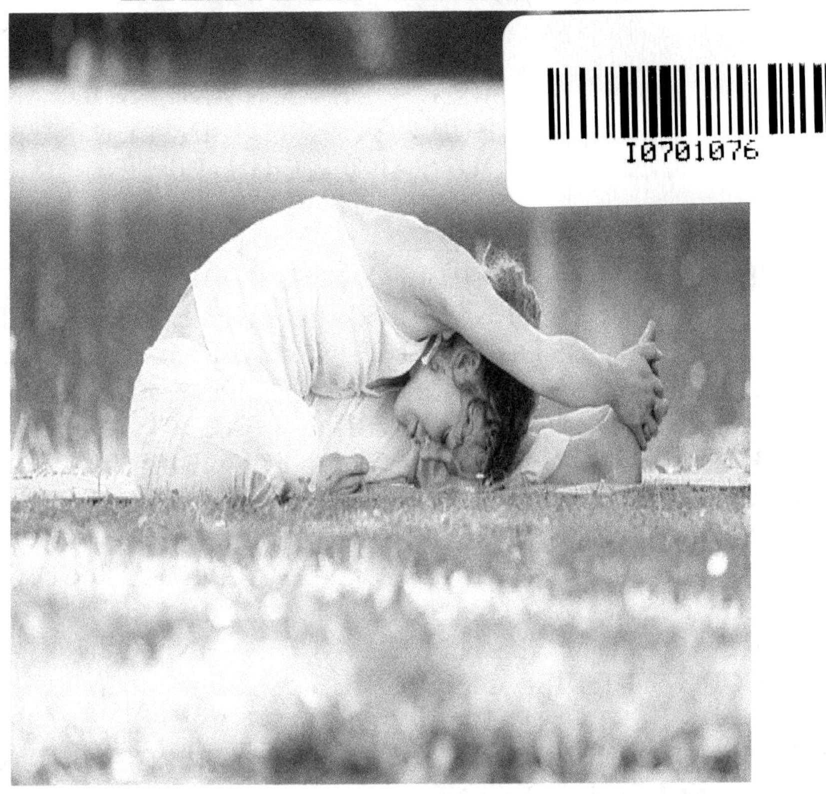

Small Steps to a Healthier You
Peter McAllen

TABLE OF CONTENT

1.0 INTRODUCTION TO EXERCISE AND FITNESS

1.1 OVERVIEW OF FITNESS AND EXERCISE

Fitness and exercise are essential for promoting general health and wellbeing. They can significantly affect both our psychological and physical well-being and are vital parts of a healthy lifestyle. This chapter will examine the value of fitness and exercise, define these terms, and talk about how they affect our general health.

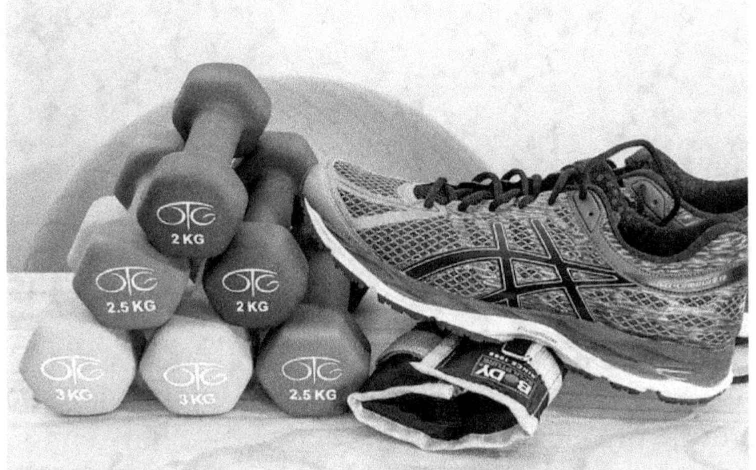

What Exercise Means

Any repetitive, structured, and planned physical activity with the aim of enhancing or preserving physical fitness is considered exercise. It's an all-encompassing term that covers everything from weight lifting and jogging to yoga and dancing.

The FITT theory, which stands for frequency, intensity, time, and type, is an essential component of exercise.

Exercise frequency, exercise intensity, exercise length, and exercise type are all related to how frequently and what kind of exercise you perform. One particular workout routine that applies the FITT principle would be jogging three times a week for thirty minutes each time.

What Fit Is

Being physically active, mentally focused, and emotionally stable are the characteristics of fitness. It is frequently determined by a person's capacity to carry out regular duties and activities without experiencing excessive fatigue. Being able to lift large weights or run a marathon is not the only measure of fitness.

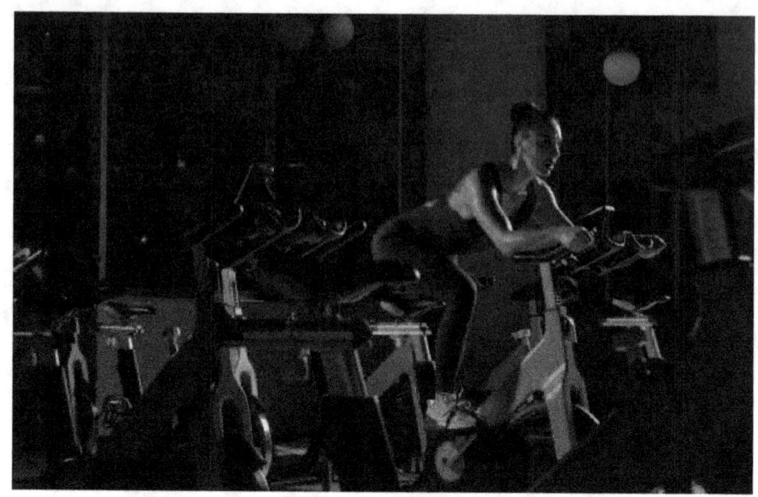

Fitness is made up of a number of elements, such as flexibility, physical strength, cardiovascular endurance, and body composition. To build and maintain each of these elements—which are essential to total fitness—different forms of exercise are needed.

1.2 THE VALUE OF FITNESS AND EXERCISE

Maintaining a healthy body weight, lowering the risk of chronic illnesses like cancer, diabetes, and heart disease, and enhancing general quality of life all depend on exercise and fitness. Frequent exercise can also aid elevate mental health, lessen stress and anxiety, and boost mood.

To sum up, fitness and exercise are essential components of a healthy lifestyle and are critical for preserving general health and wellbeing. We may enhance our physical and mental well-being and live better lives by realizing the benefits of fitness and exercise and implementing them into our everyday routines.

Advantages of Frequent Exercise

There are numerous advantages to regular physical activity for both our physical and mental health. The benefits of maintaining an active lifestyle are varied and profound, ranging from elevating our mood to bettering our general health. We will examine the many advantages of consistent physical activity in this section, along with the reasons it is essential to upholding a healthy lifestyle.

Enhanced Heart Wellness

A major advantage of consistent exercise is better cardiovascular health. Exercises that increase heart rate, like jogging, cycling, or brisk walking, strengthen the heart muscle, reduce blood pressure, and enhance blood flow. Thus, the chance of heart disease, stroke, and other cardiovascular diseases is decreased.

Control of Weight

Being physically active on a regular basis is essential for managing weight. It promotes muscular growth and calorie burning, both of which are crucial for keeping a healthy weight. Furthermore, exercise increases metabolism, which facilitates weight management and helps avoid obesity.

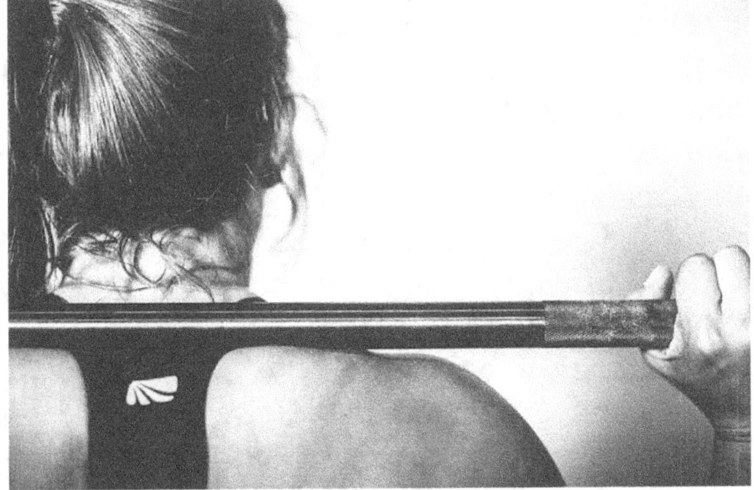

Higher Mental Well-Being

Mental health is significantly impacted by physical activity. It elevates mood, lessens the signs of anxiety and despair, and enhances mental health in general. Endorphins, sometimes known as "feel-good" hormones, are released when exercise is performed and have the potential to reduce stress and elevate mood.

Enhanced Endurance and Strength of Muscles

Regular exercise, particularly strength training activities, can assist build muscle strength and endurance. By doing this, you not only increase your capacity to carry out daily duties but also lower your chance of injury and perform better physically overall.

Improved Balance and Flexibility

Stretching exercises combined with regular exercise can help increase balance and flexibility. This is particularly crucial as we get older since it can keep us mobile and independent while reducing the risk of falls.

Improved Quality of Sleep

Sleep quality has been demonstrated to be enhanced by physical activity. Regular exercise can improve your sleep quality, help you fall asleep more quickly, and lessen the chance that you'll wake up in the middle of the night. This may result in a more revitalizing and pleasant night's sleep.

Enhanced Immune Response

Engaging in regular physical activity can boost your immunity, reducing your vulnerability to common ailments like the flu and colds. White blood cells and antibodies are produced more readily when one exercises, and they are vital for warding off diseases.

Augmented Cognitive Capacity

Increased cognitive function and a lower risk of cognitive deterioration have been associated with physical activity.

Frequent exercise helps lower the chance of acquiring neurodegenerative disorders like Alzheimer's disease and improve memory, attention, and decision-making abilities.

In summary, engaging in regular physical activity has numerous advantages for our mental and physical well-being. We may raise our mood, control our weight, strengthen our cardiovascular system, and generally improve our quality of life by making regular exercise a part of our daily routines.

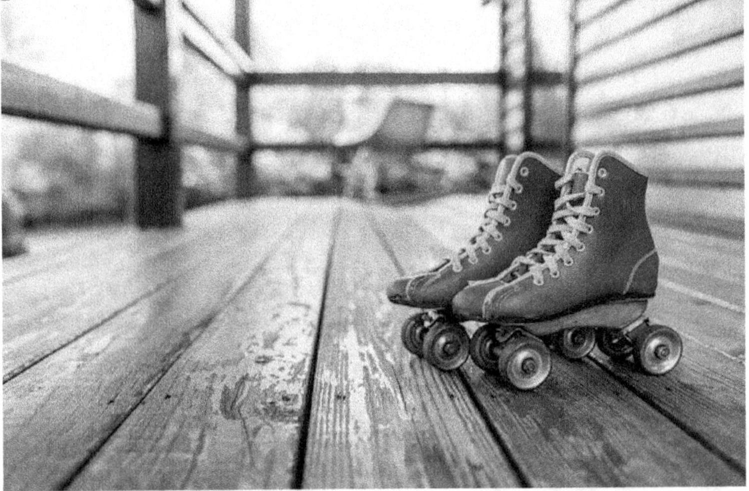

1.3 AN OVERVIEW OF THE VARIOUS EXERCISE TYPES

There are many different types of physical activity, and each has special advantages for our bodies and minds. You may design a well-rounded fitness program that fits your requirements and goals by being aware of the various workout options. We'll go over a few common workout categories here, such as aerobic, strength, flexibility, and balance activities.

Exercises for the Heart

Exercises that raise your heart and breathing rates are referred to as cardiovascular exercises, or aerobic exercises. These workouts are great for building endurance, burning calories, and strengthening the heart. Cardiovascular exercises encompass many activities such as walking, jogging, cycling, swimming, and dance. You can perform these exercises at different intensities based on your fitness level and objectives.

Exercises for Strength Training

The goals of strength training activities are to increase muscle tone, strength, and endurance. These workouts put your muscles to the test by employing resistance, like weights or resistance bands. Strength exercise can enhance overall body composition, speed up metabolism, and increase lean muscle mass. Exercises with weights, bodyweight exercises (such as squats and push-ups), and resistance band workouts are common ways to build strength.

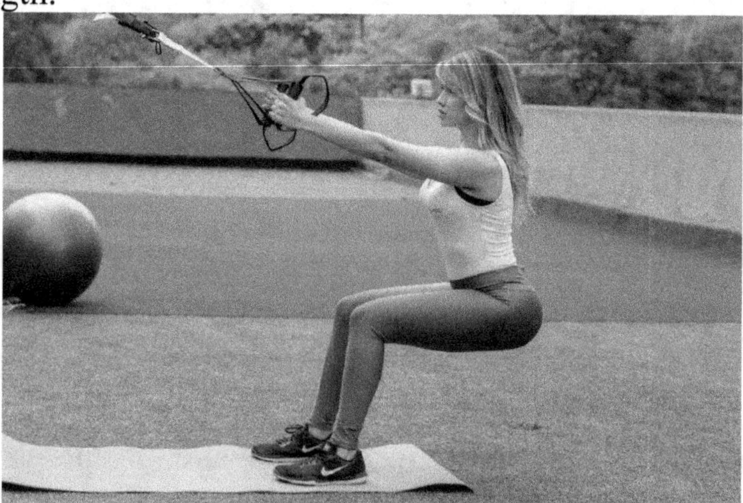

Exercises for Flexibility

Stretching activities, commonly referred to as flexibility exercises, assist in increasing joint flexibility and range of motion. These exercises can lessen tense muscles, enhance posture, and assist avoid accidents. Stretching techniques for improving flexibility include yoga, dynamic stretching, and static stretching. To preserve or increase flexibility, frequent flexibility exercises are necessary.

Exercises for Balance

Exercises that improve balance are essential for reducing falls and enhancing stability, particularly as we age. These workouts support the development of stronger muscles related to balance and coordination. Heel-to-toe walking, balance board exercises, and standing on one leg are a few examples of balancing exercises. You can lower your chance of falling and enhance your general balance by including balancing exercises in your routine.

1.4 DIFFERENT EXERCISE TYPES

Apart from the primary classifications stated previously, numerous other forms of physical activity might enhance your general well-being. Among them are:

- Functional training aims to increase general functioning by emphasizing motions that resemble daily tasks.
- High-intensity interval training (HIIT), which switches between brief rest intervals or lower-intensity workouts and short bursts of vigorous exercise.
- Pilates, which emphasizes flexibility, strength in the core, and general body training.
- Tai Chi, a style of martial arts that places an emphasis on deliberate, slow motions to enhance mental health, flexibility, and balance.

- Group exercise courses that provide an enjoyable and social approach to stay active, including aerobics, spinning, or Zumba.

In summary, you can develop a well-rounded level of fitness by including a range of exercises in your fitness regimen. You can enhance your general health, fitness level, and quality of life by combining aerobic, strength training, flexibility, and balancing exercises.

Exercise's Significance for General Health

Exercise is vital to general health and well-being; it's not only about looking nice or reducing weight. Engaging in regular physical activity can have a significant positive effect on our bodies and minds, resulting in greater health and a higher standard of living. This section will discuss the value of exercise for general health and the reasons that everyone should make it a priority in their lives.

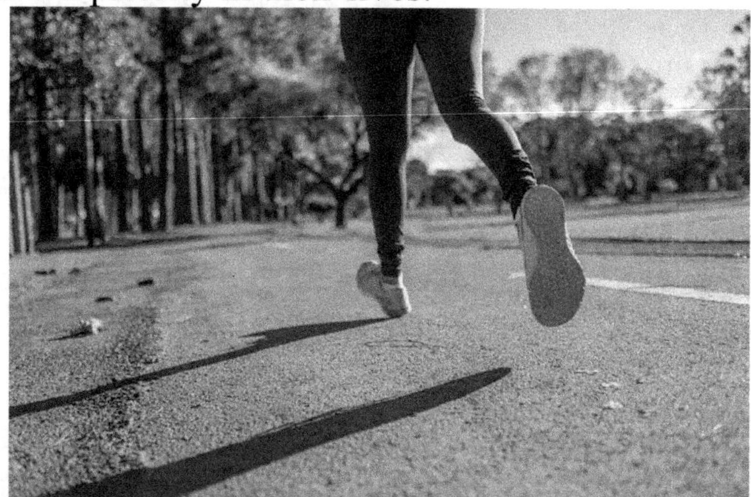

Advantages for Physical Health

There are several advantages to regular exercise for physical health. It improves cardiovascular health and lowers the risk of heart disease, stroke, and high blood pressure by strengthening the heart and lungs .Maintaining a healthy weight is essential for preventing obesity and its associated diseases, including type 2 diabetes and several cancers. Exercise also plays a major part in this process. Exercise also contributes to increased muscle flexibility and strength, which can improve overall physical performance and lower the chance of injury.

Advantages for Mental Health

Exercise is good for your physical and mental health in addition to your physical health. Endorphins are neurotransmitters released during physical activity that increase sensations of happiness and wellbeing. This can lessen stress, anxiety, and depressive symptoms while elevating mood in general. Enhancement of cognitive function through exercise has also been connected to enhanced memory, concentration, and decision-making abilities.

Enhanced Life Quality

Exercise on a regular basis can greatly enhance quality of life. It can boost vitality, enhance general wellbeing, and improve the quality of sleep. Because it gives one a sense of mastery and success, physical activity can also increase confidence and self-esteem. Furthermore, because exercise promotes social interaction and connection, it can help lessen feelings of loneliness and isolation.

Age and Longevity

It has been demonstrated that exercise lengthens life and encourages healthy aging. Frequent exercise can aid in the prevention of aging-related chronic conditions like osteoporosis, arthritis, and cognitive decline. In addition to preserving our freedom and mobility as we age, exercise enables us to keep living life to the fullest.

Prevention of Diseases

One effective strategy for preventing disease is exercise. It can lessen the chance of getting long-term illnesses like heart disease, type 2 diabetes, and some cancers. The immune system is strengthened by exercise, which aids in the body's ability to fend against diseases and infections.

To sum up, physical activity is crucial for general health and wellbeing. It has numerous advantages for both physical and mental health, enhances life quality, encourages long life and healthy aging, and aids in the prevention of chronic illnesses. You may have a happier, healthier, and more satisfying life by prioritizing exercise.

2.0 CARDIOVASCULAR EXERCISES FOR HEART HEALTH.

2.1 AN EXPLANATION OF CARDIOVASCULAR EXERCISES

Exercises that raise your heart and breathing rates are referred to as cardiovascular exercises, or aerobic exercises. The cardiovascular system, which includes the heart, lungs, and blood arteries, is the main objective of these activities. They are necessary to preserve general fitness and heart health.

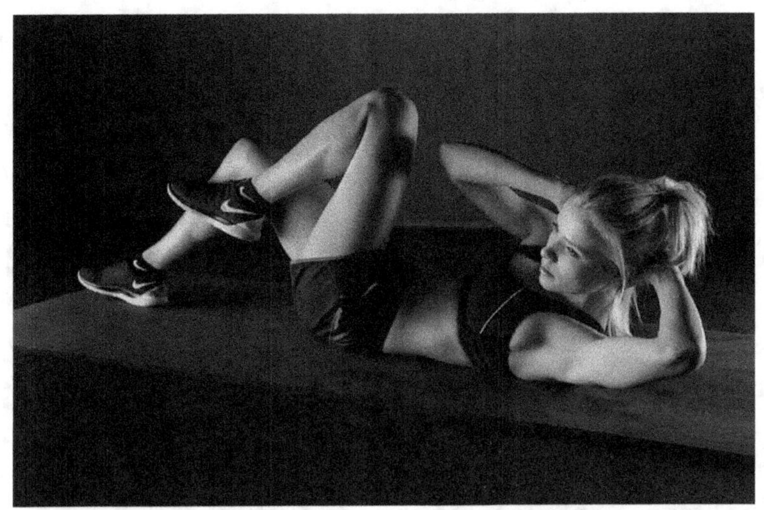

Your heart generates more blood during cardiovascular exercise in order to supply oxygen to your muscles. Your heart and lungs will function more efficiently as a result of the increased blood flow. Your resting heart rate can be lowered and your cardiovascular endurance can be increased with consistent cardiovascular exercise.

Cardiovascular exercise comes in different forms, with intensities ranging from low to high. Low-intensity workouts are good for novices or people with mobility concerns because they are easy on the joints, such as walking or light cycling. Exercises that are moderate in intensity, such as swimming or running, raise your respiratory and heart rates and present a greater cardiovascular strain. Running and HIIT (High-Intensity Interval Training) are examples of high-intensity exercises that push your body to its limits and provide the greatest cardiovascular benefits.

Exercises involving the heart have many other health benefits than heart health improvement. They can aid in weight management by decreasing body fat and burning calories. Because they expand lung capacity and strengthen respiratory muscles, they also enhance lung function.

Cardiovascular workouts can also improve your mental and emotional well-being. Endorphins are brain chemicals released during physical activity that have the dual benefits of improving mood and acting as natural painkillers. Frequent exercise has been associated with a decrease in stress, anxiety, and depressive symptoms.

It's not too difficult to include cardiovascular exercises in your routine. To make exercising more fun, pick things you enjoy doing, like dancing, hiking, or sports. Aim for 75 minutes of intense activity spaced out throughout the week, or at least 150 minutes of moderate-intensity aerobic activity per week.

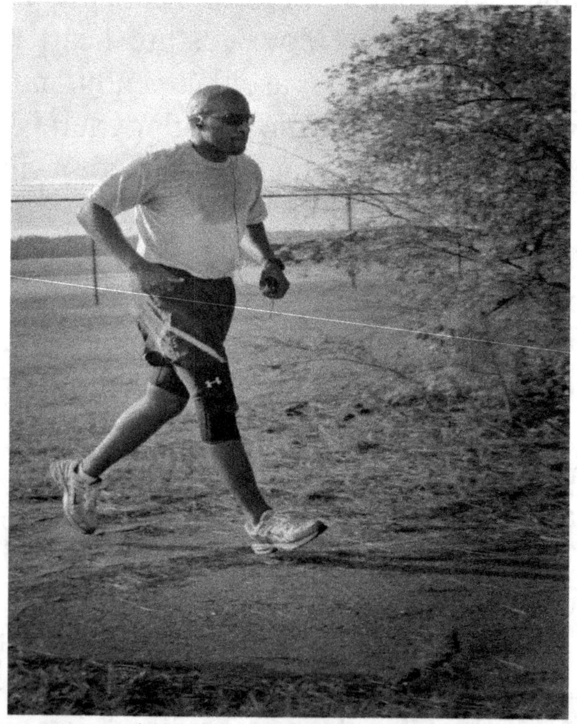

It's important to begin cautiously, particularly if you haven't worked out in a while or are new to it. As your fitness improves, start with shorter sessions and progressively increase the length and intensity. Always pay attention to your body's signals, and cease if you feel any pain or discomfort.

Cardiovascular activities are essential for preserving heart health and general wellbeing, to sum up. Numerous advantages are provided by them, such as increased cardiovascular endurance, better weight management, and mood enhancement. You may make major progress toward living a healthier lifestyle by adding these activities to your schedule.

2.2 ADVANTAGES FOR CARDIOVASCULAR HEALTH

Since the heart is an essential organ that pumps blood and oxygen throughout the body, heart health is key to general well-being. Participating in heart-healthy activities can significantly improve your longevity and quality of life. The following are some important advantages of keeping your heart healthy:

1 . **Lower Risk of Cardiovascular Disease** : Eating a well-balanced diet and engaging in regular physical activity can help reduce the risk of heart disease, which includes disorders including coronary artery disease, heart attacks, and strokes. Engaging in these activities contributes to the maintenance of good blood pressure, cholesterol, and blood sugar levels—all of which are heart disease risk factors.

2. **Enhanced Cardiovascular** Endurance: By strengthening the heart muscle, cardiovascular activities improve the heart's ability to pump blood more effectively.

This enhances overall endurance and lessens tiredness by boosting circulation and oxygen delivery to the muscles and organs.

3. Weight Management : You can maintain a healthy weight or reduce extra weight by getting regular exercise. Obesity and excess weight raise the risk of heart disease and place additional strain on the heart. You can attain and maintain a healthy weight, which will lessen the strain on your heart, by eating a balanced diet and remaining active.

4. Improved Mental Health and Mood : Research has indicated that physical activity can lessen anxiety and depressive symptoms as well as enhance mood. Endorphins are naturally occurring brain chemicals that are released during physical activity and have a positive effect on mood. Enhancing your emotional well-being also lowers your chance of experiencing stress-related cardiac problems.

5 . Enhanced Energy: Engaging in regular exercise helps minimize symptoms of exhaustion and increase your energy levels. Your muscles can work harder and longer without becoming fatigued when your heart is in good health and functioning well. This is because a healthy heart can better supply oxygen and nutrients to your muscles.

6. Better Sleep : Exercise helps control your sleep cycles and enhance the quality of your sleep. Reduced risk of heart disease and other chronic illnesses has been associated with improved sleep.

7 . Stress Reduction: Getting some exercise will help you feel less stressed and tense. It lessens the synthesis of stress chemicals like cortisol by promoting physical and mental relaxation. Reducing stress can be beneficial to heart health.

8 . **Extended Lifespan** : By keeping your heart in good condition with regular exercise and a well-balanced diet, you can extend your life expectancy and lower your chance of dying young from heart-related conditions.

In summary, putting heart health first through regular exercise, a balanced diet, and stress reduction can have a number of positive effects, such as lowered risk of cardiovascular disease, enhanced mood, better sleep, and longer life spans. You can extend your life and improve your health by implementing these behaviors into your everyday routine.

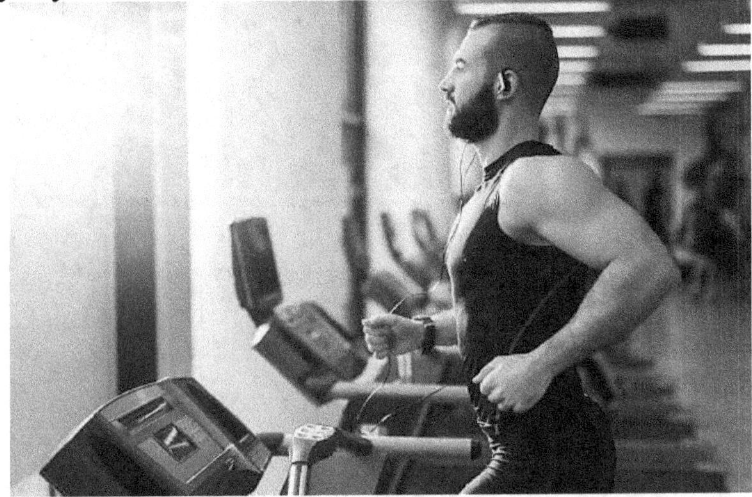

2.3 CARDIOVASCULAR EXERCISE EXAMPLES INCLUDE JOGGING, SWIMMING, AND ENDURANCE

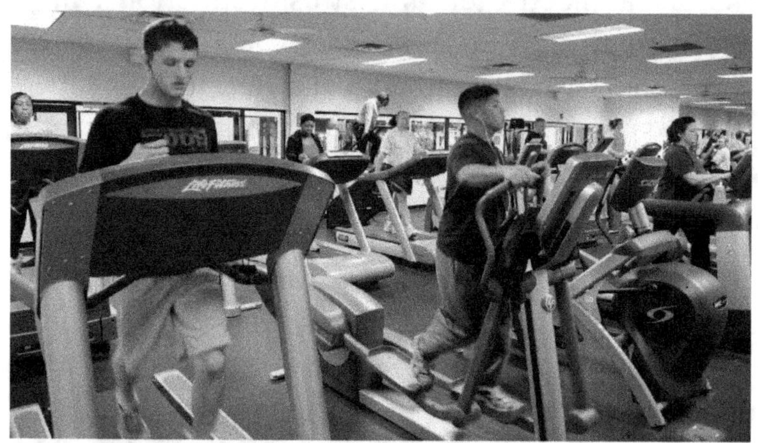

There are many different types of cardiovascular exercise; the important thing is to choose ones you will love and be able to stick with. Here are a few well-known cardiovascular workout examples:

1. Running: Increasing your heart rate and cardiovascular endurance can be achieved through running. Running is a flexible and efficient cardiovascular workout, whether you choose to jog in your neighborhood or take to the trails in a local park.

2. Swimming : This full-body, low-impact activity works your entire body. It's extremely advantageous for those who have joint problems or are searching for a revitalizing form of exercise. Whether you swim in broad water or just laps in a pool, swimming can strengthen your cardiovascular fitness

3. Riding a bike: Riding a road or mountain bike outside or indoors on a stationary cycle is another great cardiovascular workout. Cycling is a terrific way to explore the outdoors or get to work while strengthening your leg muscles and improving your cardiovascular health.

4 . Walking: You can work your cardiovascular system simply and effectively practically anyplace with walking. Walking is an excellent approach to enhance heart health, whether you walk briskly around your neighborhood or make walking a part of your daily routine, like taking the stairs or going to work.

5. Dancing: Increasing your heart rate and cardiovascular fitness with dancing is enjoyable. Dancing may be a terrific way to stay healthy and have fun at the same time, whether you take dancing classes or just dance around your living room.

6. Jumping Rope : Enhancing your cardiovascular endurance and coordination, jumping rope is a high-intensity cardiovascular workout. It's an excellent, almost anytime exercise that raises your heart rate immediately.

7. Rowing : Working the legs, core, and upper body, rowing is a great cardiovascular workout. Whether you row in a class or on a machine at the gym, rowing may be a tough and efficient cardiovascular exercise.

8. Elliptical Training : This low-impact cardiovascular exercise targets the upper and lower body and is done on an elliptical machine. It's a fantastic substitute for cycling or running for those who have joint problems.

There are several other activities that might enhance your heart health; these are only a few examples of cardiovascular exercises. To get the benefits of cardiovascular exercise, it's important to pick activities you enjoy and can fit into your daily schedule.

2.4 - HOW TO INCLUDE AEROBIC ACTIVITIES IN A FITNESS PROGRAM

Cardiovascular activities must be a part of your fitness plan to maintain heart health and overall fitness. The following guidance may help you include cardiovascular activities in your program:

1. Set Reasonable Goals : To begin, decide on reasonable objectives for your cardio workout. Take into account your schedule, degree of fitness at the moment, and any health issues. Over time, try to progressively increase the length and intensity of your workouts.

2. Pick Fun Activities : Picking enjoyable activities can help your cardiovascular exercise regimen last. Find activities you enjoy doing, whether it's swimming, cycling, dancing, hiking, or running.

3. Mix It Up: Vary your cardiovascular exercises to avoid boredom and target different muscle groups. You could, for instance, run one day, swim the next, and then cycle the following day. Additionally, this type can aid in preventing overuse injuries.

4. Find a Workout Partner : Engaging in cardiovascular exercise with a friend or family member can increase your enjoyment and motivation. Along with accountability, having a workout partner increases the likelihood that you'll follow through on your plan.

5. Plan Your Workouts : Make sure to schedule your cardiovascular exercises into your calendar, just like you would any other important appointment. This can assist in ensuring that you prioritize your health and carve out time for exercise.

6. Begin Slowly : To prevent injury, start slowly if you've never done cardiovascular exercise before or if you haven't been active in a long. As your fitness increases, progressively increase the duration and intensity of your workouts from shorter, less intensive ones.

7. Warm Up and Cool Down : To get your muscles and cardiovascular system ready for exercise, warm up before beginning any cardiovascular workout. Stretch lightly to increase flexibility and help reduce discomfort in your muscles after your workout.

8. Listen to Your Body: Observe how exercise makes your body feel both during and after. In the event that you feel pain, lightheadedness, or any other worrisome symptoms, cease exercising and get medical attention.

9. Stay Hydrated: To stay hydrated and support optimal bodily function, sip on lots of water prior to, during, and following your cardiovascular exercises.

10. Monitor Your Progress : Record the length, level of intensity, and nature of your cardiovascular exercises. This can support your goal-achieving motivation by allowing you to track your advancement.

Including cardiovascular physical activity in your fitness regimen will help you become more fit overall, enhance your heart health, and elevate your mood. You may design a cardiovascular workout regimen that is both sustainable and beneficial for you by using the advice in this article.

3.0 STRENGTH TRAINING

3.1 A COMPREHENSIVE GUIDE TO MUSCLE HEALTH

Exercise that focuses on developing and strengthening muscles is called resistance training, or strength training. Strength training, on the other hand, aims to increase muscular size, strength, and endurance rather than just the cardiovascular system.

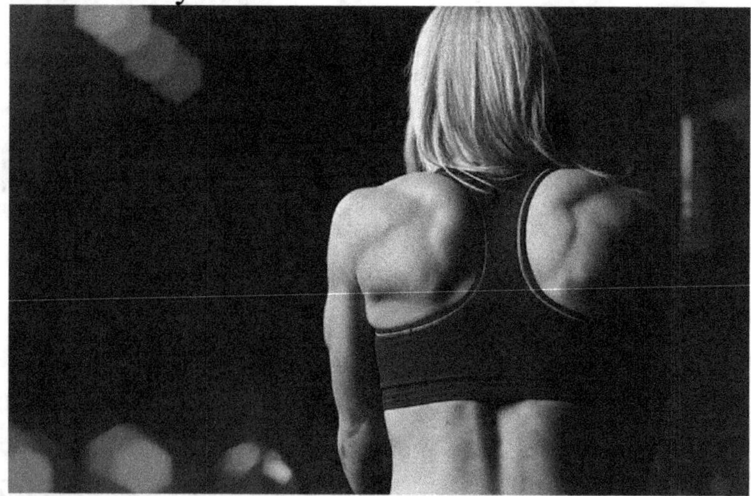

Strength training is essentially working your muscles with resistance. This resistance can come from your own body weight as well as free weights (barbells, dumbbells), weight machines, and resistance bands. In order to promote strength and muscle growth, the objective is to progressively overload the muscles, which entails steadily raising the resistance or intensity of the workout over time.

Specificity is one of the main tenets of strength training, meaning that the exercises you do should be tailored to the muscles you want to target and the results you want to accomplish. For instance, you may do exercises like squats, lunges, or leg presses if you want to improve your leg muscles. You might perform workouts like push-ups, pull-ups, or shoulder presses to focus on your upper body.

Beyond only helping you gain muscle, strength training has many other advantages. It can increase bone density, which is particularly crucial as you get older to avoid osteoporosis. Additionally, it can assist increase joint flexibility and health, which lowers the chance of injury and increases mobility all around.

Furthermore, strength exercise can help your metabolism function better. Because muscle tissue has a higher metabolic activity than fat tissue, gaining muscle may cause your metabolism to rise and enable you to burn more calories even when you're at rest. Both general health and weight management may benefit from this.

Strength training can also enhance your general quality of life by facilitating the completion of everyday chores. A strong and functional body may help you live life to the fullest, whether you're playing with your kids or grandkids, lifting groceries, or doing the laundry.

It's vital to remember that strength training should be performed carefully and correctly to prevent injuries. In order for your muscles to rebuild and become stronger in between workouts, you must also give them enough time to rest and recover. A well-rounded strength training regimen should consist of a range of exercises that focus on various muscle groups, done two to three times a week, separated by one day off.

Strength training offers numerous advantages for both physical and mental health, making it an important part of any well-rounded fitness regimen. Strength training can assist you in reaching your objectives, whether they want to gain muscle, improve your health, or improve your quality of life.

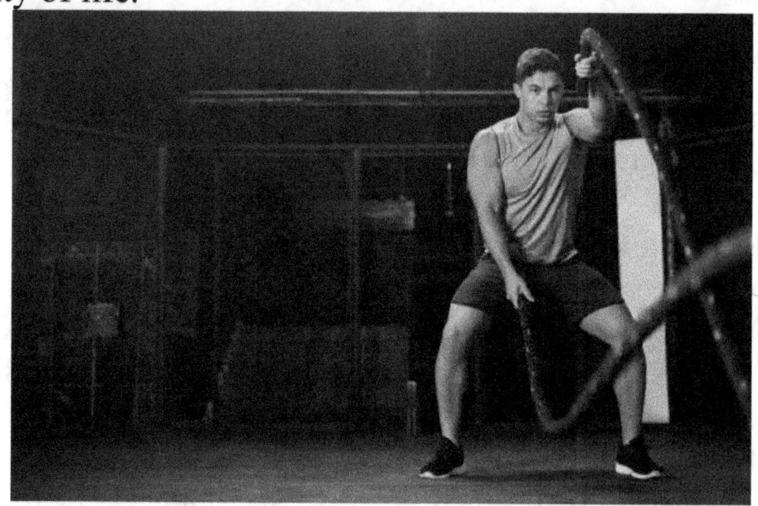

3.2 BENEFITS FOR MUSCLE STRENGTH AND ENDURANCE

Muscle strength and endurance are crucial for performing everyday activities and maintaining overall health. Strength training, which focuses on building muscle strength and endurance, offers a range of benefits that can improve your quality of life.

One of the primary benefits of strength training is increased muscle mass and strength. As you engage in regular strength training exercises, your muscles adapt by becoming larger and stronger. This increased muscle mass can improve your ability to perform tasks that require strength, such as lifting heavy objects or climbing stairs.

Strength training also improves muscle endurance, which is the ability of your muscles to sustain repeated contractions over time. This can be particularly beneficial for activities that require sustained effort, such as running a marathon or playing a long game of tennis. By improving muscle endurance, you can delay fatigue and perform better for longer periods.

In addition to enhancing muscle strength and endurance, strength training can also improve your overall physical performance. Whether you're an athlete looking to improve your performance in a specific sport or simply want to stay active and fit, strength training can help you achieve your goals.

Prevention of injuries is another advantage of strength training. You can lower your risk of sprains and strains as well as increase joint stability by building stronger muscles. This is especially crucial as you become older since imbalances and weakness in your muscles can make falls and other injuries more likely.

Additionally, strength exercise can benefit your metabolism. Because muscle has a higher metabolic activity than fat, having more muscle can increase your resting-state calorie burn. This may help with managing weight and general health.

Strength training also helps to maintain healthy bones. Similar to muscles, bones get stronger under the strain of strength exercise. This can lessen the chance of developing osteoporosis, a disorder marked by fragile and weak bones, and help prevent bone loss.

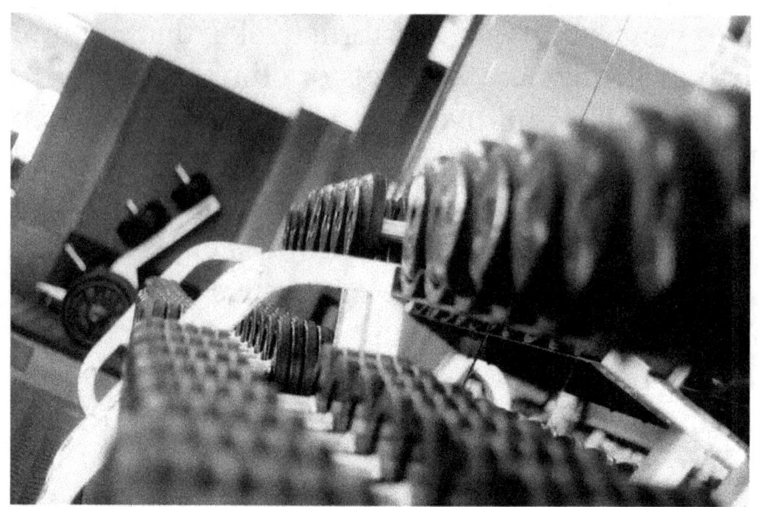

Additionally, strength exercise might benefit your mental well-being. It has been demonstrated that exercise, particularly strength training, improves mood and lessens the symptoms of anxiety and depression. Endorphins, which are endogenous substances in the brain that function as natural analgesics and mood enhancers, may have contributed to this in part.

To put it simply, strength training has numerous advantages for both general health and wellbeing and muscle strength and endurance. Strength training can help you increase the strength and endurance of your muscles, lower your chance of injury, and perform better physically in general.

3.3 WORKOUTS THAT BUILD STRENGTH INCLUDE BODYWEIGHT WORKOUTS AND WEIGHTLIFTING.

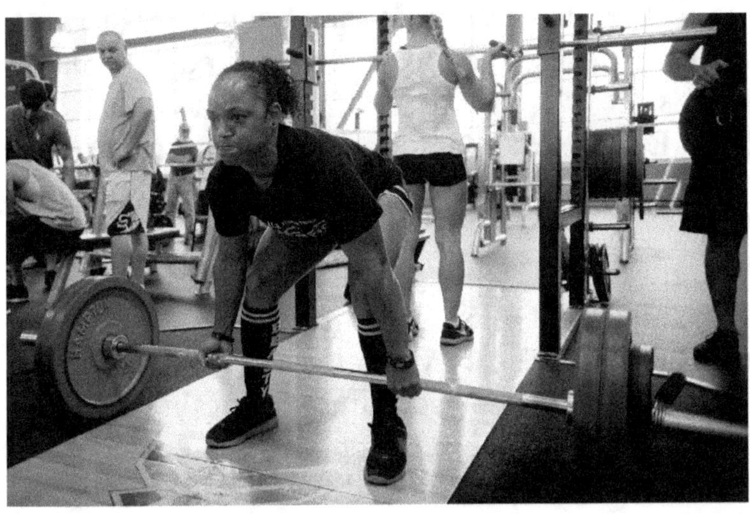

Exercises for strength training can take many different forms, but the important thing is to pick ones that can be tailored to your fitness level and target different muscle groups. These are a few well-known instances of strength training activities:

1. Weightlifting: Often referred to as resistance training, weightlifting is a traditional strength training technique in which weights are lifted in order to increase muscular mass and strength. For weightlifting exercises, you can use weight machines or free weights like dumbbells or barbells.

2. Bodyweight Exercises : Bodyweight exercises involve using your own body weight as stimulus during strength training sessions. Exercises like planks, lunges, squats, and push-ups are examples. These activities are an excellent method to develop strength without the need for any equipment and can be done anywhere.

3. Resistance Band Exercises : Resistance bands can offer resistance in a variety of directions, making them an adaptable tool for strength training. Exercises like leg extensions, lateral raises, and bicep curls can be done using resistance bands.

4. Kettlebell Exercises: A range of strength training exercises may be performed with kettlebells, which are weighted balls with handles. Kettlebell exercises that assist increase strength and flexibility include Turkish get-ups, goblet squats, and kettlebell swings.

5. Medicine Ball Exercises: Medicine balls are exercises that combine strength and coordination training using weighted balls. To enhance core strength and coordination, try medicine ball workouts like wall balls, Russian twists, and overhead slams.

6. Exercises with Resistance Machines : In gyms, resistance machines are a common option for strength training. For exercises like leg presses, lat pulldowns, and chest presses, these machines use weighted plates or cables as resistance.

7. Plyometric Exercises: These high-intensity workouts can enhance your power and speed. Burpees, box jumps, and jump squats are a few examples of exercises that can assist increase muscle strength and agility.

8. Isometric workouts : In order to develop strength, isometric workouts need maintaining a stationary position. Static lunges, wall sits, and planks are a few examples of exercises that can assist increase muscle stability and endurance.

9. Circuit Training : Using little to no pause in between, a succession of strength training exercises is performed during a circuit training session. This can assist in increasing muscle strength and endurance as well as cardiovascular health.

10. Functional Training: To increase strength and flexibility for daily activities, functional training focuses on exercises that replicate common movements. Exercises like push-ups, lunges, and squats are a few examples that can enhance general functional fitness.

To obtain a well-rounded strength training regimen, you can target different muscle groups by incorporating a range of these exercises into your routine. As you advance, keep in mind to start out slowly, practice good technique, and progressively increase the weight and intensity.

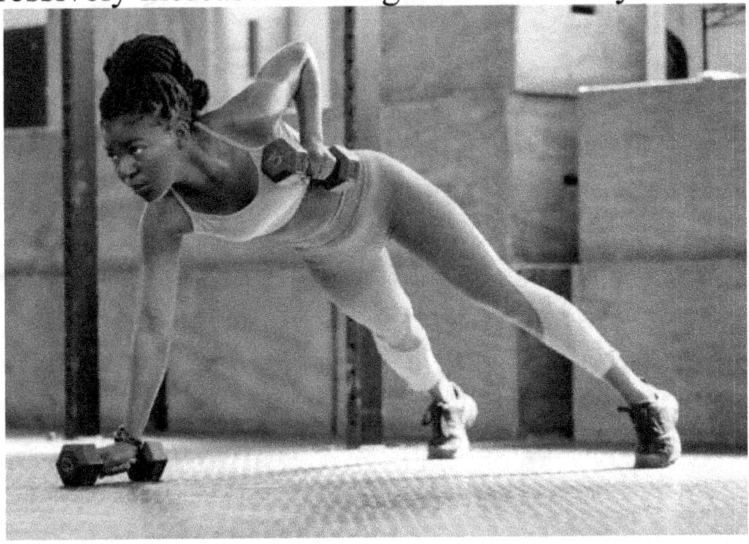

3.4 HOW TO BEGIN A STRENGTH-TRAINING ROUTINE SAFELY

There are a few important things to take into account before beginning a strength training regimen. Strength training may be right for you if you speak with a healthcare provider or fitness expert first, especially if you have any health issues. In order to give your muscles and joints time to adjust, it's important to begin slowly with modest weights or resistance bands. For the purpose of avoiding injuries and maximizing the benefits of your exercise, concentrate on acquiring correct form and technique.

To improve blood flow to your muscles, warm up with gentle aerobic or dynamic stretches before each workout. To increase your comfort and safety, wear supportive shoes and weightlifting gloves, among other appropriate equipment. Over time, increase the resistance, weight, or intensity of your workouts to make incremental progress. Exercise should be stopped if you feel pain, discomfort, or unusual weariness. Pay attention to your body.

In order to promote muscle growth and regeneration, give yourself enough time to recover between workouts. To help you recover after strength training and support your efforts, eat a balanced diet and drink enough water. Keep a log of your workouts, including the exercises, sets, repetitions, and weights utilized, to track your improvement. To keep pushing your muscles and prevent plateaus, make any necessary adjustments to your regimen.

You can begin a strength training program safely and successfully by following these rules, which will enhance your general health and fitness.

4.0 STRETCH AND FLEXIBILITY FOR MOBILITY

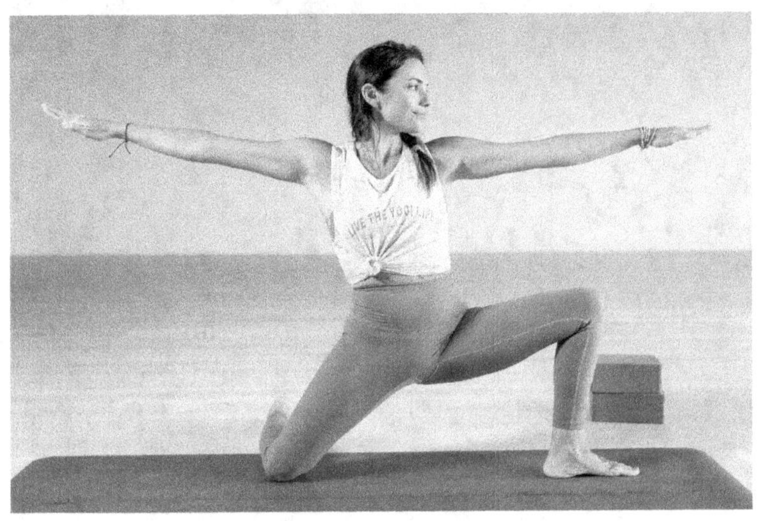

4.1- THE VALUE OF FLEXIBILITY FOR GENERAL FITNESS

Although it's frequently disregarded, flexibility is an essential part of general fitness. It describes how well your muscles and joints can move across their whole range of motion. Good flexibility can lower your risk of injury and enhance your balance, coordination, and posture.

Improved joint health is one of flexibility's main advantages. Your joints can move more freely and are less likely to become stiff and painful when they are flexible. This is especially crucial as you become older since as people age, their flexibility tends to decline, increasing their risk of falls and injuries.

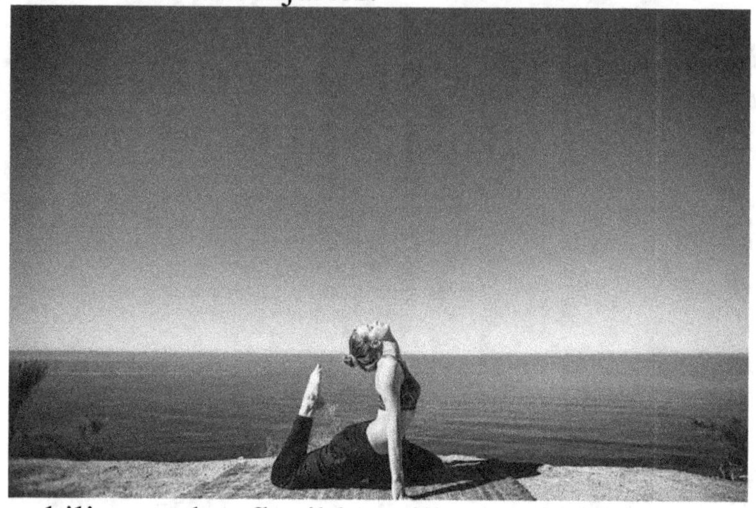

Your ability to be flexible will also help you perform better in sports. Whether you're a weightlifter, dancer, or runner, being flexible can improve your performance and lower your chance of injury. For instance, having flexible shoulders can help you carry weights overhead, and having flexible hamstrings will help you run with a better stride.

Furthermore, flexibility might help you have better posture by letting your muscles stretch and unwind. Numerous problems, such as headaches, neck pain, and back pain, can be brought on by poor posture. You can assist in resolving these concerns and lowering the likelihood of more complications by strengthening your flexibility.

An additional advantage of flexibility is enhanced circulation. Stretching improves blood flow to your muscles, which can lessen pain and hasten the healing process after a workout. By encouraging improved circulation throughout your body, this increased blood flow can help enhance your general health.

Maintaining a healthy level of mobility in your joints also requires flexibility. Your joints may stiffen and lose some of their range of motion as you age, making daily tasks more challenging. You can keep your joints mobile and healthy as you age by being flexible, which will keep you active and self-sufficient.

It's not too difficult to include flexibility exercises in your workout regimen; you don't need any specialized equipment to perform them anyplace. Exercises for improving flexibility include Pilates, yoga, and stretching. Your general level of fitness, flexibility, and posture can all be enhanced by these workouts.

In summary, flexibility is a crucial aspect of total fitness that shouldn't be disregarded. It can enhance range of motion, circulation, posture, sports performance, and joint health. You can lower your chance of injury and enhance your general health and well-being by including flexibility exercises in your program.

4.2 -ADVANTAGES OF STRETCHING EXERCISES

There are numerous advantages to stretching exercises for the body and mind. Stretching can assist increase general well-being, decrease muscle stress, and improve flexibility in your everyday routine.

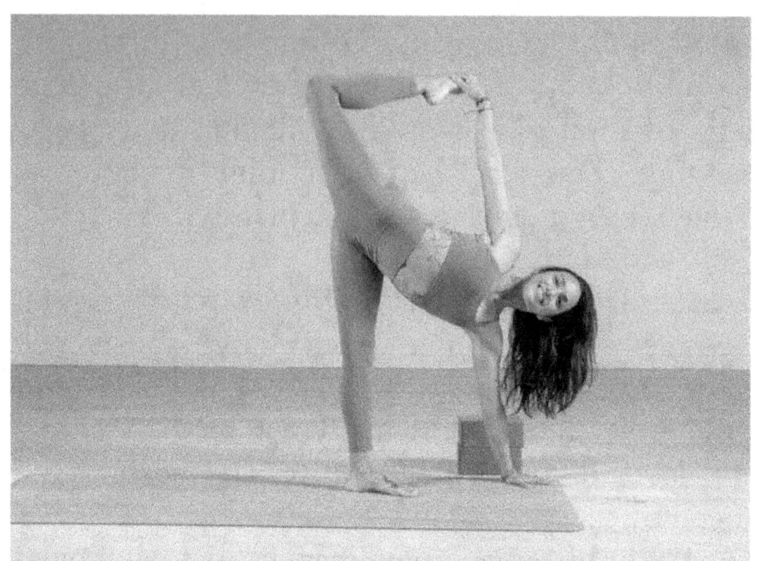

More flexibility is one of the main advantages of stretching exercises. Stretching facilitates the entire range of motion of joints by lengthening muscles and tendons. Increased flexibility can make daily tasks easier and more comfortable, improve sports performance, and lower the chance of injury.

Stretching techniques can also aid in easing stiffness and tension in the muscles. Tight muscles can restrict your range of motion and make you more vulnerable to injury. Stretching lowers the chance of strains and enhances general muscle function by assisting in the relaxation and release of tension from the muscles.

Stretching exercises can also enhance blood flow to the muscles and circulation. This enhanced blood flow can support the health of the muscles overall and aid in the delivery of nutrients and oxygen to the muscles, facilitating their recovery from exercise.

Moreover, stretching can aid with posture by extending tense muscles that can be causing the body to become misaligned. Frequent stretching will help address postural abnormalities and lower your chance of shoulder, neck, and then back pain.

Stretching activities can improve mental health in addition to their physical effects. Stretching can aid in lowering bodily tension and stress levels while fostering a calm and relaxed attitude. Stretching is an excellent exercise to include in your daily routine since it can also aid with concentration and focus.

Exercises that stretch the muscles also help with balance and mobility. Our muscles tend to get tighter as we get older, which affects our balance and mobility. Stretching can help maintain and increase flexibility, which enhances mobility and balance and lowers the chance of accidents and falls.

Exercises that increase range of motion and flexibility can also help athletes perform better. Athletes may move more effectively and efficiently with increased flexibility, which can improve their performance in any of the sports they engage in.

Stretching exercises are quite simple to incorporate into your regular routine and don't require any additional equipment to be performed anywhere. Static stretches, dynamic stretches, and yoga positions are a few types of stretching exercises. These exercises are appropriate for people of all fitness levels since they may be customized to target particular muscle groups or regions of tightness.

There are several advantages to stretching exercises for the body and mind. Stretching can help you become more flexible, relieve stress in your muscles, increase circulation, correct posture, and improve your general well-being. Stretching exercises can be a useful addition to any fitness program, whether you're an athlete wanting to improve performance or a non-athlete looking to relieve stress and increase mobility.

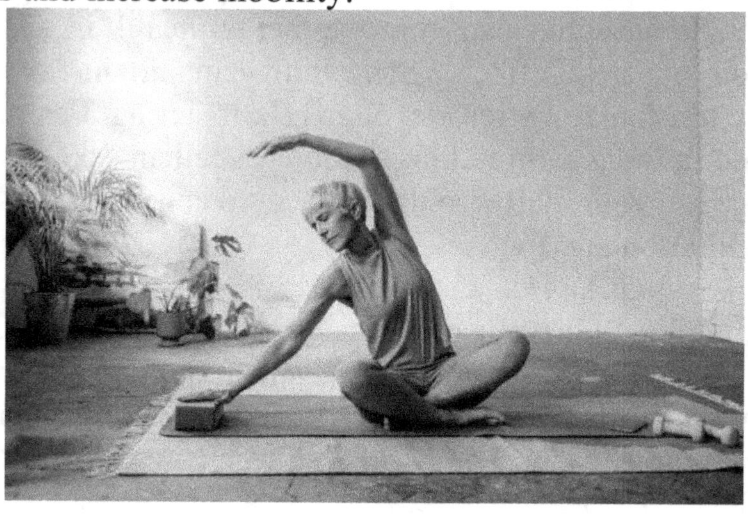

4.3 - EXAMPLES OF STRETCH PRACTICES, YOGA, PILATES, AND OTHER FORMS OF FLEXIBILITY EXERCISES

Exercises for flexibility can take many different forms, and mixing things up in your routine will help you work on different muscle groups and increase your overall flexibility. These are a few well-known instances of flexibility exercises:

1. **Yoga** : Yoga is a physical posture, breathing, and meditation practice that enhances strength, flexibility, and mental clarity. There are numerous variations of yoga, from calming and easy to strenuous and demanding. Asanas, or yoga positions, concentrate on strengthening and balancing the body while simultaneously extending and stretching the muscles.

2. Pilates: Pilates is a type of exercise that emphasizes flexibility, posture correction, and basic muscle strengthening. Pilates is a great option for increasing flexibility and body awareness because its workouts frequently call for exact alignment and controlled movements.

3. Stretching Exercises : You can modify your stretching exercises to focus on particular muscle groups or tight spots. Stretching statically—that is, holding a stretch for a while—can assist increase range of motion and ease tense muscles. Moving through a range of motion during dynamic stretching can assist increase flexibility and warm up the muscles before working out.

4. Tai Chi: Tai Chi is a slow-moving Chinese martial technique that also incorporates meditation and deep breathing. Tai chi can help with stress reduction and relaxation, as well as flexibility, balance, and coordination.

5. Dancing: Participating in dance courses or routines that call for movement and stretching can be a fun method to increase flexibility. Stretches that can increase range of motion and flexibility are frequently used in dance forms like jazz, ballet, and contemporary dance.

6. Foam Rolling : Foam rolling is a self-myofascial release technique that helps alleviate tense muscles and increase flexibility. Applying pressure on tense muscles with a foam roller can help relieve tension and increase range of motion.

7. Resistance Band Exercises : A range of stretching exercises that increase flexibility can be done using resistance bands. For instance, you can stretch your hips, shoulders, or hamstrings with a resistance band.

8. Gymnastics: Adding some exercises with a gymnastics theme to your activities might assist increase flexibility, even though gymnastics may not be for everyone. Backbends, splits, and bridges are a few exercises that can assist increase general mobility and flexibility.

9. Martial Arts: As part of their training, martial arts styles like jiu-jitsu, taekwondo, and karate frequently include stretches. These workouts can enhance agility, balance, and flexibility.

10. Water-Based Exercises: Swimming and aqua aerobics are two exercises with little impact when it comes to increasing flexibility. In addition to providing for mild stretching, the water's resistance can aid in muscular strengthening.

Adding a range of flexibility exercises to your regimen will help you become more flexible overall, relax your muscles, and increase your level of fitness. To improve flexibility and preserve general health, select activities that you enjoy and can regularly incorporate into your routine, regardless of your preference for yoga, Pilates, stretching routines, or other forms of flexibility exercises.

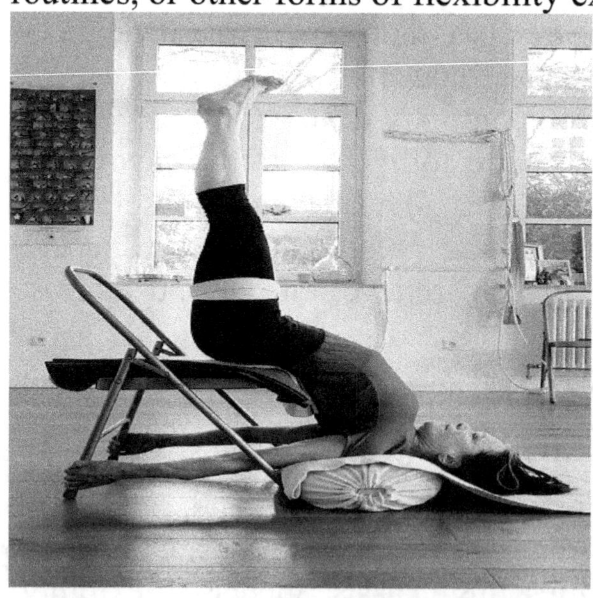

4.4 - HOW TO INCREASE RANGE OF FLEXIBILITY AND AVOID GETTING HURT

A vital component of preserving general health and fitness is increasing flexibility and avoiding injuries. While injury prevention involves lowering the risk of strains, sprains, and other ailments that might happen during physical exercise, flexibility refers to your muscles' and joints' ability to move through their complete range of motion.

Warming up correctly before exercise is a crucial step towards increasing flexibility and reducing the risk of injury. Your muscles become more pliable and less prone to damage with increased blood flow following a thorough warm-up. Dynamic stretches, which require you to move your muscles through their whole range of motion, are crucial to incorporate into your warm-up.

Frequent stretching is also necessary to increase range of flexibility and lower the chance of injury. Static stretches, which include holding a stretch for a while, can help increase flexibility and lengthen muscles. All of the major muscle groups should be stretched, including the ones that are frequently overlooked, such the calves, hip flexors, and hamstrings.

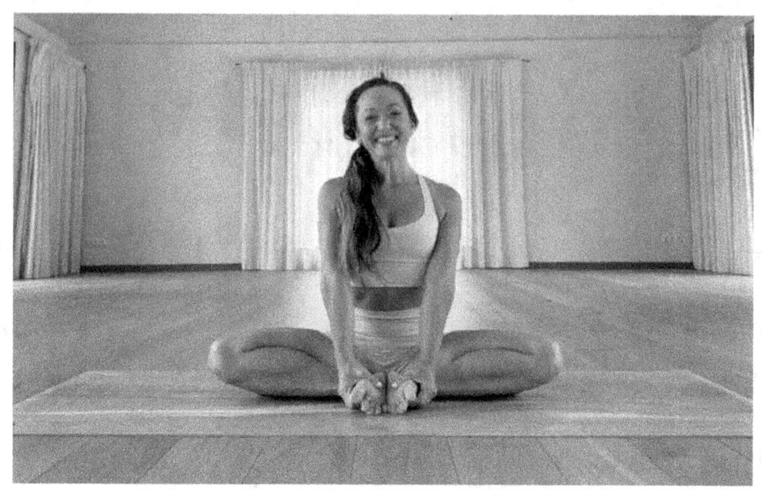

It's essential to stretch with good form to avoid damage. Steer clear of bouncing or jerking motions as these might cause muscular tension. Rather, concentrate on deliberate, steady motions that progressively lengthen the stretch. When you experience any severe or sharp pain, pay attention to your body and stop.

Another crucial element in increasing flexibility and reducing the risk of injury is staying hydrated. Maintaining sufficient water intake lowers the chance of injuries and cramping while also preserving muscular elasticity. Throughout the day, especially before and after activity, sip on lots of water.

Including different stretching methods in your regimen might also help you become more flexible. Proprioceptive neuromuscular facilitation (PNF) stretches, which combine contracting and relaxing the muscles to increase flexibility, can be among the dynamic, static, and other types of stretches.

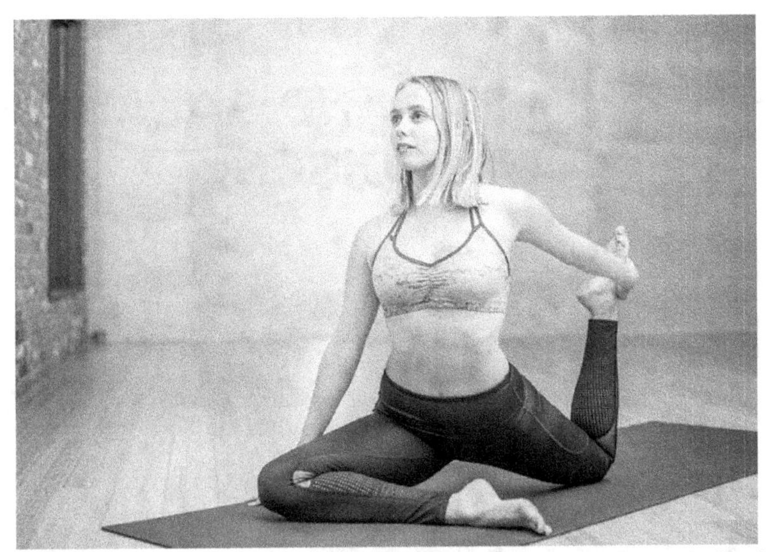

The secret to increasing flexibility and avoiding injuries is to go slowly. As your flexibility increases, start with stretches that are comfortable and work your way up to longer or more intense poses. Overexertion can result in damage, so pay attention to your body's needs and move forward at a speed that suits you. It's also crucial to keep your flexibility regimen balanced. Make sure to stretch every major muscle group, even the ones that are frequently overlooked. This can lessen the chance of injury and assist avoid muscular imbalances.

Finally, maintaining general health and fitness requires both increasing flexibility and avoiding injuries. You can increase flexibility, lower your risk of injury, and improve your general well-being by warming up correctly, stretching frequently, using proper form, staying hydrated, incorporating a variety of stretching techniques, progressing gradually, and maintaining balance when performing your flexibility routine.

5.0 STABILITY AND BALANCE EXERCISES

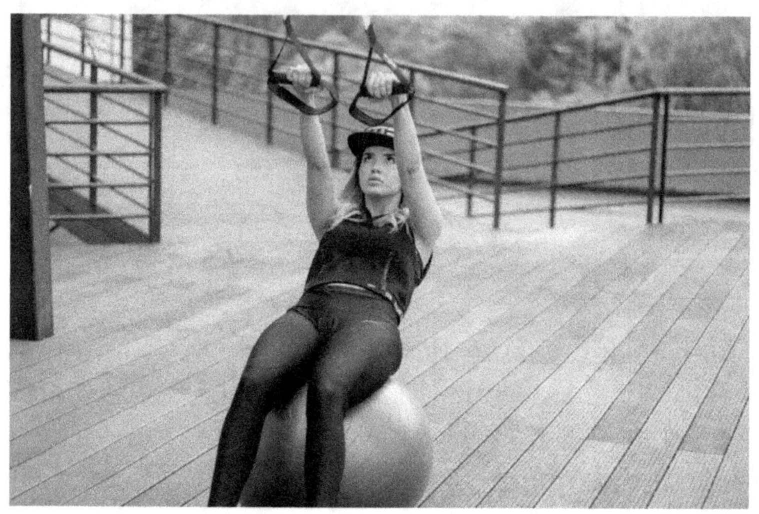

5.1 THE VALUE OF STABILITY AND BALANCE FOR DAY-TO-DAY TASKS

To carry out daily tasks with confidence and ease, one needs balance and stability. Having strong balance and stability can assist prevent falls and injuries when you're walking, standing, or reaching for something. This is especially true as you get older.

Enhanced coordination is one of the main advantages of balance and stability exercises. You may move more effectively and efficiently by strengthening the muscles that govern balance and movement with the help of these exercises. Everyday activities like walking, climbing stairs, and carrying goods might feel easier and more natural with improved coordination.

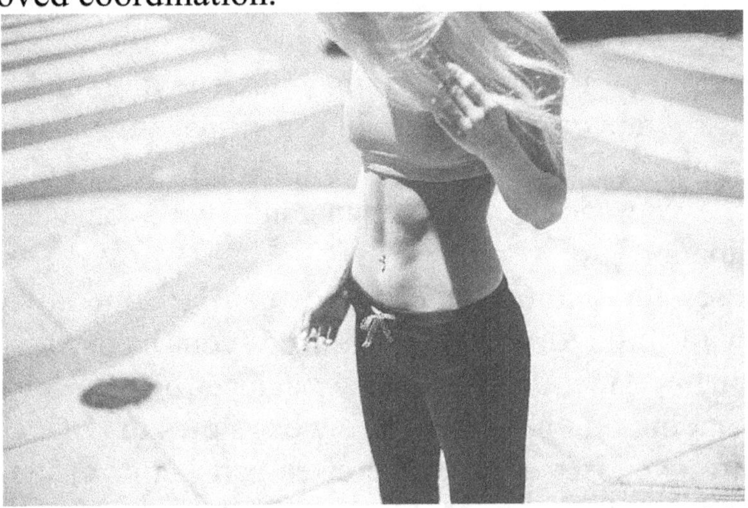

Exercises for stability and balance can also aid with posture. Maintaining normal spine alignment and lowering the risk of shoulder, neck, and back pain depend on having good posture. You can assist correct your posture and lower your chance of developing postural imbalances by strengthening the muscles that support your spine and enhancing your balance.

Exercises for stability and balance can also aid in enhancing proprioception, or the body's awareness of its own position in space. Due to the age-related decrease in proprioception, this may be very helpful for elderly individuals. You can lower your chance of falling and increase your level of mobility and independence by strengthening your proprioception.

Enhanced athletic performance is an additional advantage of balance and stability workouts. Professionals and weekend warriors alike can benefit from improved stability and balance, which can improve their performance in sports and other physical activities. Your total athletic ability, agility, and response time can all be enhanced by these activities.

Exercises for stability and balance can also aid in the prevention of injuries. You may lessen your chance of sprains, strains, and other injuries that might happen during physical activity by strengthening the muscles that support your joints and enhancing your balance and coordination.

Exercises for stability and balance can be done anywhere and with little difficulty, provided you have the right equipment. Heel-to-toe walks, balance board exercises, and standing on one leg are a few examples of balance and stability exercises. These exercises can help you become more stable and balanced, lower your chance of falling and getting hurt, and generally live a better, more fulfilling life. Ultimately, stability and balance are necessary for carrying out daily tasks with confidence and ease. You may enhance your sports performance, posture, proprioception, coordination, and injury prevention by including balance and stability exercises in your regimen. Exercises for balance and stability can be beneficial for everyone, whether they are young athletes trying to improve their performance or older adults looking to retain their independence.

5.2 THE ADVANTAGES OF BALANCE TRAINING IN REDUCING THE RISK OF INJURIES

Any fitness program must include balanced activities, but this is especially true for older persons who may be more likely to fall. By enhancing balance, coordination, and stability, these activities can lessen the chance of injury and assist prevent falls. The following are some main advantages of balanced exercise for preventing falls:

1. Better Balance: Among the main advantages of balanced exercise is better balance. By strengthening the muscles involved in balance and coordination, these exercises help to preserve stability and reduce the risk of falling.

2. Improved Coordination: The capacity to carry out flexible, deliberate motions is known as coordination, and it is bolstered by balanced workouts. You may move more quickly and effectively and lower your chance of tripping or stumbling by increasing your coordination.

3. Enhanced Stability : Enhanced stability is an additional advantage of balanced exercise. Particularly in the ankles, knees, and hips, these exercises help to strengthen and stabilize the muscles that support your joints. This can act as a strong support base, preventing falls.

4. Reduced likelihood of Falling : The lower risk of falls is possibly the biggest advantage of balanced exercise. Especially for older folks, you may dramatically lower your chance of tripping, slipping, or falling by increasing your stability, balance, and coordination.

5. Enhanced Confidence : Balanced exercise can also help bolster confidence, particularly in senior citizens who might be afraid of falling. You can gain more self-assurance in your capacity to walk safely and freely by strengthening your balance and stability.

6. Maintained Independence : Loss of independence is one of the major effects of falls, especially for older persons. You can lower your chance of falling and prolong your period of independence by doing balanced workouts.

7. Improved Movement : Exercises that are balanced can also aid in enhancing movement in general. You may move more freely and easily and continue to be active and involved in everyday activities by developing your balance, coordination, and stability.

8. Better Posture: By fortifying the muscles that support the spine, balanced workouts can also aid in the improvement of posture. Maintaining balance and preventing falls need proper posture.

9. Improving Entire Health : Taking part in well-rounded exercise might benefit your general well-being. These workouts can strengthen muscles, lower the chance of developing chronic illnesses like diabetes and hypertension, and enhance cardiovascular health.

10. Decreased Risk of Injury : Lastly, balanced exercise can assist in lowering the chance of getting hurt in falls and other mishaps. You can move more securely and effectively and lower your chance of sprains, strains, and other injuries by increasing your balance, coordination, and stability.

Any fitness regimen must include balanced activities, but this is especially true for senior citizens who want to be independent and avoid falling. These exercises can help lower the risk of falls, increase confidence and independence, and improve general health and well-being by enhancing balance, coordination, and stability.

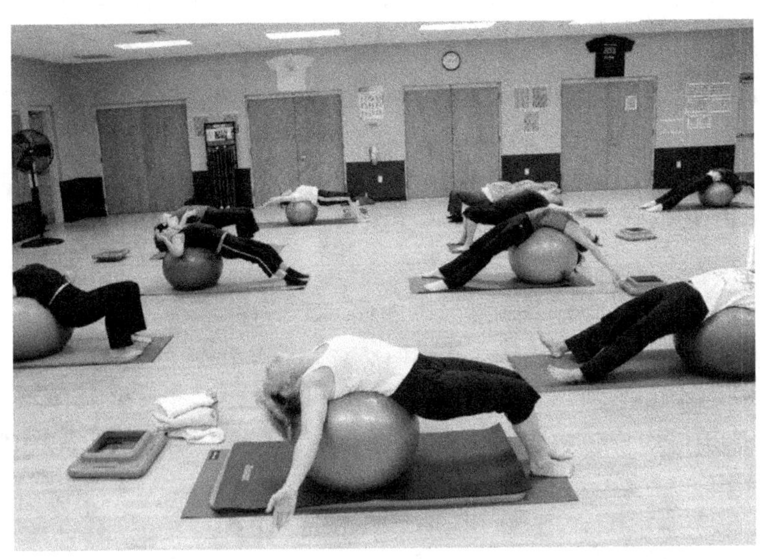

5.3 EXAMPLES OF STABILITY AND BALANCE EXERCISES.

Balance and stability exercises are essential for improving overall stability, decreasing falls, and improving coordination. Examples of balance and stability exercises are as follows:

1. Tai Chi: Tai Chi is a gentle martial art that stresses slow, purposeful movements and deep breathing. It can especially benefit the elderly by improving their balance, flexibility, and coordination.

2. Balance Board Exercises : Using a balance board, wobble board, or balancing disc will help you improve your balance and stability by challenging your proprioception and core muscles. These exercises can be as easy as standing on the board and keeping your balance, or they can be more difficult like lunges and squats.

3. One-Leg Stands: This exercise might help with balance and stability. Start with one leg and stand for ten to thirty seconds, then switch to the other leg. As you improve, you can try harder variants like closing your eyes or moving your arms, or you can increase the duration of the hold.

4. Heel-to-toe walks : In this exercise, you walk in a straight line, putting the heel of one foot in front of the toes of the other with each step. This is a balance and coordination workout that you may do outside or indoors.

5. Chair Yoga: Chair yoga is the practice of yoga poses while seated or with a chair for support. It's ideal for those who struggle with mobility or are new to exercising because it can help with strength, flexibility, and balance enhancements.

6. Standing Leg Swings: This exercise involves swinging the other leg back and forth while standing on one leg. With this exercise, you may improve your hip range of motion, flexibility, and balance.

7. Side Leg Raises : This kind of exercise involves raising one leg out to the side while standing on the other. This workout strengthens the hips and improves stability and balance.

8. Bosu Ball Exercises : A Bosu ball, a half-ball balance trainer, can be used for a variety of stability and balance exercises. Examples of exercises you can do with the Bosu ball include squats, hand pushups, and one-footed standing.

9. Plank Variations : Plank exercises help strengthen the core, which is important for balance and stability. To make it harder to maintain your balance, try a plank with your hands or forearms, or place your feet or hands on a balancing board.

10. Stability Ball Exercises: Using a stability ball can help with balance and stability by using the core muscles of the body. Two examples include sitting on a ball with one foot raised off the ground and performing push-ups with both hands on the ball.

By including these balance and stability exercises into your routine, you may improve your coordination, balance, and stability, which will reduce your risk of falling and improve your quality of life overall.

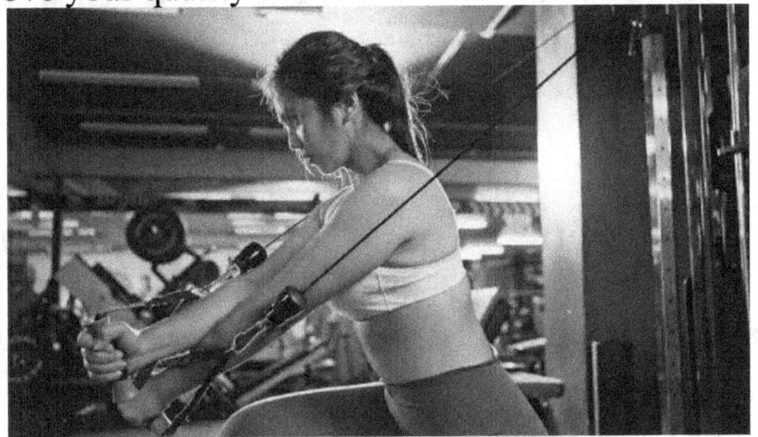

5.4 - HOW TO INTEGRATE BALANCING EXERCISES INTO YOUR EXERCISE ROUTINE

If you want to improve your stability, balance, and coordination, you need to incorporate balanced exercises into your workout routine. These exercises can lower the chance of falling, enhance athletic performance, and enhance overall quality of life.

Here are some pointers for integrating balanced workouts into your fitness regimen:

1. have clear Goals : It's important to have clear goals before including balanced activities into your routine. Decide on your objectives, such as enhancing balance, boosting stability, or preventing falls. Setting measurable, specific goals will help you stay motivated and track your progress.

2. Start cautiously: If you've never done balanced exercise before, start out slowly to avoid overdoing it and getting harmed. Easy exercises like one-leg stands and board balancing are a good place to start. As you gain comfort, gradually increase the time and intensity.

3. Mix It Up: Include a variety of well-balanced activities in your program to keep things interesting and give your body different challenges. Try doing some different activities like Pilates, Tai Chi, or yoga if you want to improve your balance, stability, and coordination.

4. Pay Attention to Form : When performing balanced exercises, excellent form is crucial to ensuring you're working the right muscles and reducing your risk of injury. To guarantee your safety and optimal performance, pay special attention to your alignment, posture, and breathing throughout each exercise.

5. Combine with Other Exercises : A more all-encompassing fitness regimen that also includes balanced activities might integrate cardiovascular, strength, and flexibility exercises. You may create a well-rounded fitness program by mixing different workout techniques with balanced activities.

6. Be Consistent: As with any other form of exercise, consistency is key when including balanced exercises into your routine. Try to perform balance exercises two or three times a week to help with stability, coordination, and balance.

7. Pay Attention to Your Body : Pay attention to how your body feels throughout and after a well-rounded workout. If you experience any pain or discomfort, stop working out immediately and get help from a doctor if necessary.

8. Modify as Needed: If you have any physical limitations or health concerns, modify the balanced activities to suit your needs. If you have trouble standing, you could try doing balancing exercises while seated.

9. Stay inspired : At times, it might be challenging to find the motivation to incorporate well-rounded activities into your routine. Set small, manageable goals, reward yourself when you reach new heights, and find a group or training partner to hold you accountable.

10. Track Your Improvement : Keep a journal of your workouts and record any improvements you see in your coordination, stability, or balance. Acknowledge your successes and use setbacks as opportunities to learn and adjust your program as needed.

Adding comprehensive exercises into your fitness routine can improve your overall health and well-being. By setting clear goals, starting slowly, varying your routine, paying attention to form, combining with other exercises, being consistent, listening to your body, making necessary modifications, staying motivated, and keeping track of your progress, you can improve your balance, coordination, and stability as well as lead a more active and healthy lifestyle.

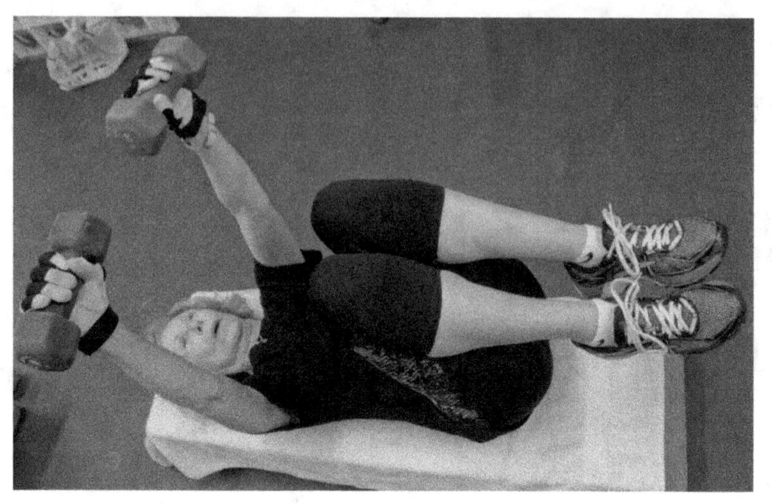

6.0 STABILITY AND POSTURE VIA CORE STRENGTH

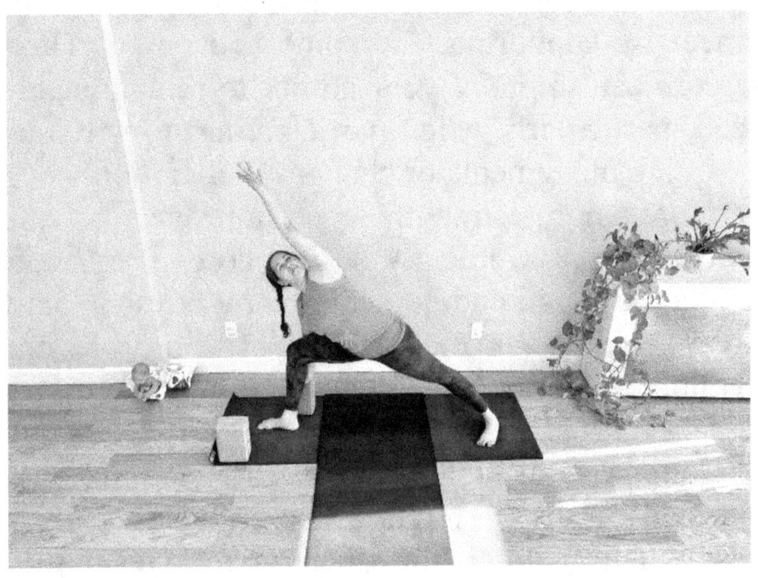

6.1 THE IMPORTANCE OF CORE STRENGTH FOR STABILITY AND POSTURE

Core strength is necessary for stability and good posture. All movements are based on the muscles of the abdomen, lower back, hips, and pelvis, which are collectively referred to as the core muscles. These muscles also support the spine.

One of the key benefits of core strength for stability and posture is better alignment. Your core muscles support your pelvis and spine, keeping you in proper alignment throughout the day. This could reduce the chance of rounding the shoulders and stooping over, which can lead to poor posture and back pain.

Core strength also plays a major role in stability. The core muscles reduce the risk of falls and injuries during movement by supporting the spine and pelvis. Having a strong core can improve your ability to remain stable and balanced, particularly when participating in activities that require quick movements or changes in direction.

Furthermore, core strength can improve an athlete's performance as a whole. A strong core is essential for strength, agility, and endurance in many physical activities and sports. Increasing the strength of your core muscles will improve your lifting, running, and leaping performance.

Doing exercises that focus on your core can improve your stability and posture. Exercises like crunches, planks, and Pilates can help build and lengthen the muscles in the core. These exercises can be customized to your fitness level and done at home or in a gym.

In addition to improving posture and stability, core strength also reduces the risk of injury. A strong core reduces the risk of sprains and strains during physical activity by stabilizing the pelvis and spine. By strengthening your core, you can improve your overall level of fitness and reduce the likelihood of injuries preventing you from participating in your favorite activities.

All things thought of, having a strong core is essential for stability, good posture, and overall health. Core-strengthening exercises can help you become more stable, reduce your risk of back pain, straighten your posture, and improve your overall performance in sports. There are several advantages to including core exercises into your regimen for your health and wellbeing, no matter how expert you are in your field.

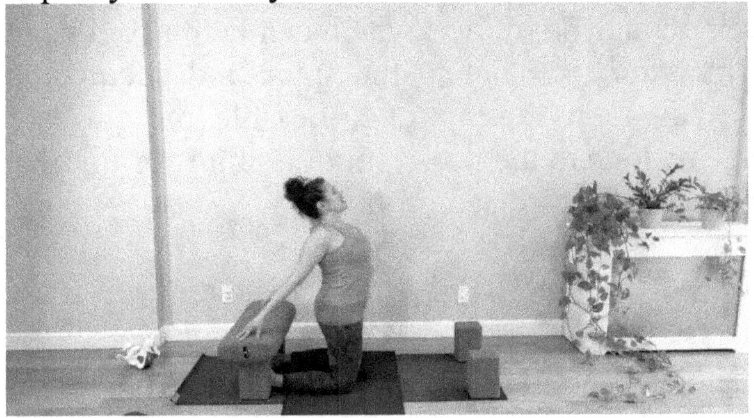

Benefits of core workouts for preventing back pain
It makes sense that core exercises are often recommended as a preventative measure for back problems. Strengthening the muscles in your abdomen, lower back, hips, and pelvis can help reduce your risk of back pain and injury by supporting your spine and improving posture.
One of the key benefits of core exercises for reducing back pain is improved spinal stability. The muscles of the core support the pelvis and spine, provide a firm foundation for movement, and lessen the likelihood of strain or injury to the muscles of the back. Strengthening these muscles can assist maintain the proper alignment of your spine and reduce the likelihood of issues like herniated discs or muscular imbalances, which can cause back pain.
Better posture is another advantage of less back pain, and core exercises help attain this. Poor posture, such as slouching or hunching over, can put additional strain on the spine and result in pain or discomfort. You may help preserve the spine's appropriate alignment and lower your

chance of developing postural problems, which can exacerbate back pain, by strengthening your core muscles. Exercises focused on the core can also assist increase general strength and flexibility, which can help avoid back problems. In order to maintain the spine and endure the stresses of daily activities, strong, flexible muscles are preferable. This lowers the possibility of strains or injuries that might result in back discomfort.

6.2 BASIC EXERCISES THAT MAY BE HELPFUL IN AVOIDING BACK PAIN

1. Planks: Including the muscles in the lower back, hips, and abdomen, planks are an excellent method of strengthening the core. Remaining in a plank posture for 30 to 60 seconds can enhance your stability and core strength.

2. Bridges: Another great exercise for stabilizing the spine and strengthening the core is the bridge. With your feet flat on the floor and your knees bent, lie on your back. Then, raise your hips off the floor by using your glute and core muscles.

3. Bird Dogs: Training with bird dogs is an excellent way to strengthen and stabilize your core.
Beggin on your hands and knees, stretch one arm and the other leg while maintaining a contracting core. After a brief period of holding, swap sides.

4. Superman : The lower back muscles are crucial for maintaining the spine and avoiding back pain, and Superman exercises can help strengthen them. Stretch your arms above while lying on your stomach. Then, raise your legs and arms off the floor by using your lower back and core muscles.

By including these exercises in your regimen, you can lessen your chance of developing back discomfort and strengthen your core muscles. To prevent overexertion, it's crucial to begin carefully and increase the duration and intensity of your workouts gradually. The best course of action if you currently have back problems or concerns is to share with an expert in the health field before starting any other exercise..

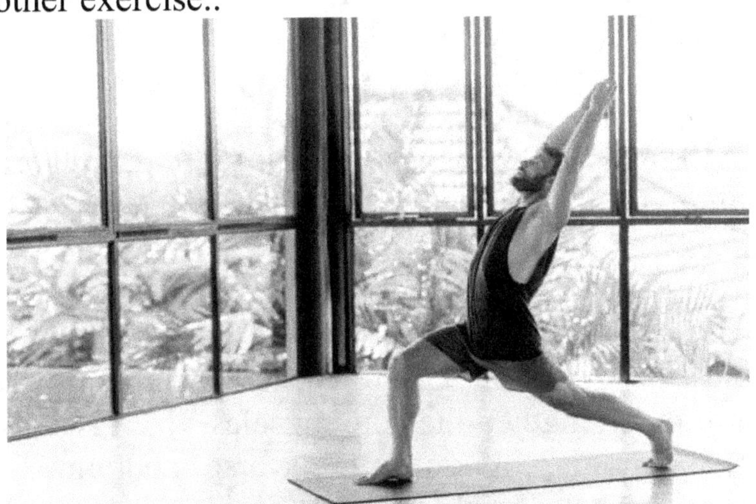

6.3 - HOW TO PROPERLY BUILD YOUR CORE MUSCLES

A mix of focused exercises, good form, and consistency is needed to properly strengthen the core muscles. To successfully strengthen the core muscles, follow these important steps:

1. Pay Attention to Form : To make sure you're targeting the right muscles and lowering your chance of injury, proper form is crucial when completing core workouts. Throughout each exercise, pay close attention to your breathing, posture, and alignment to ensure both safety and maximum efficacy.

2. Start with Basic Exercises : Planks, bridges, and bird dogs are examples of fundamental core exercises that focus on all main muscle groups. By starting with these exercises, you may strengthen your foundation before moving on to more difficult ones.

3. Progress Gradually : As you get more attuned to performing simple workouts, progressively up the ante on your workouts' complexity and intensity. This can be extending the time spent holding planks, increasing the resistance during workouts, or introducing novel variations.

4. Include Variety: It's critical to include a range of exercises that focus on various muscle groups in order to successfully strengthen the core muscles. Exercises for the rectus abdominis, obliques, transverse abdominis, and lower back muscles might be a part of this.

5. Include Functional Movements: Include exercises in your routine that are designed to replicate real-world activities, like overhead presses, lunges, and squats. These exercises strengthen and stabilize the entire body while also working the core muscles.

6. Adopt Correct Breathing Techniques: Breathing correctly can help you contract your core muscles and increase how effective your workouts are. To activate your core muscles during the exertion phase of any workout, take a deep breath and release it quickly.

7. Engage the Entire Core : During every exercise, pay special attention to activating the muscles in your belly, lower back, hips, and pelvis. This will guarantee that every muscle in the core is effectively strengthened.

8. Be Consistent : Building stronger core muscles requires consistency, just like any other type of training. To increase strength and stability, try to engage in core exercises two or three times a week.

9. Listen to Your Body : Observe how core workouts make your body feel both during and after. Should you feel any pain or discomfort, cease the workout right once and seek medical advice if needed.

10. Merge with Cardio and Strength Training: Include core exercises in a comprehensive fitness program that also focuses on strength training and cardiovascular exercise. This will increase the efficacy of your core exercises and help you become more fit overall.

These techniques can help you develop your core muscles, increase your stability, and lower your chance of injury by including core exercises into your daily routine. To get the best results, always start out cautiously, make progress gradually, and pay attention to your body.

7.0 FUNCTIONAL TRAINING

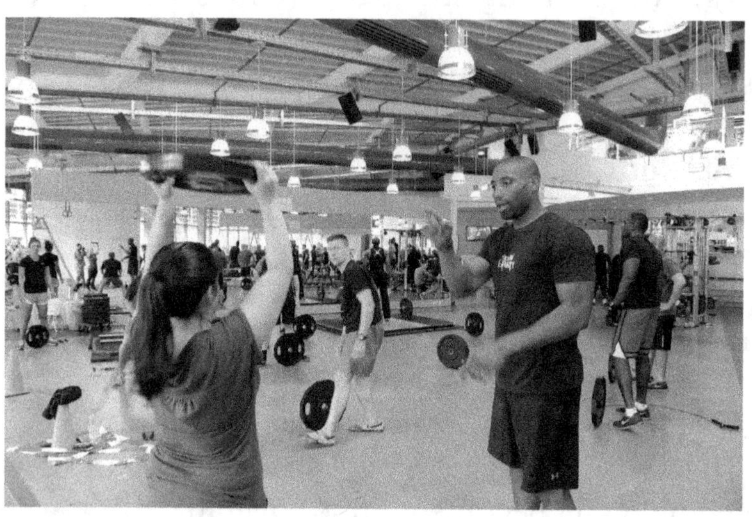

7.1 USING FUNCTIONAL TRAINING FOR DAILY ACTIVITIES

The goal of functional training is to increase the body's capacity to carry out daily tasks more securely and effectively. Functional training places more emphasis on motions that resemble everyday tasks than traditional strength training, which frequently isolates specific muscles or muscle groups. Examples of these movements include squatting, lunging, pushing, pulling, and spinning. Enhancing general functional fitness, or the capacity to carry out daily duties without difficulty or danger of harm, is the aim of functional training.

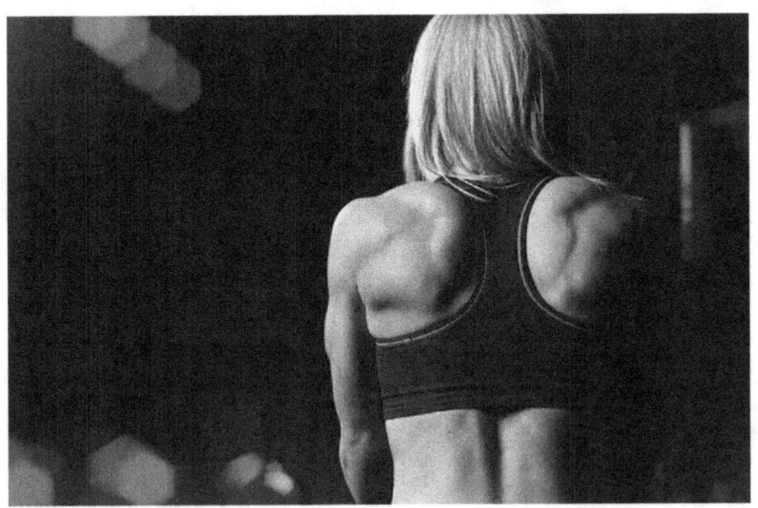

Moving beyond single muscle motions, one of the main tenets of functional training is the idea of movement patterns. For example, functional training could include workouts that entail lifting and moving objects in place of just bicep curls to strengthen the biceps because this more closely reflects a movement pattern seen in everyday life. Functional training helps enhance balance, strength, flexibility, coordination, and balance—all of which are necessary for carrying out daily tasks—by teaching movement patterns.

The utilization of multi-joint exercises, which require many muscle groups and joints to operate together, is another crucial component of functional training. Exercises of this kind more closely resemble the motions we perform on a daily basis, which frequently call for the synchronization of multiple muscle groups and joints. Examples of multi-joint exercises are lunges, deadlifts, and squats; these movements work several joints and muscle groups simultaneously.

Since a strong, stable core is necessary for carrying out daily tasks safely and effectively, functional training also places a heavy emphasis on core stability. In order to maintain good posture and alignment throughout many functional exercises, the core muscles must be engaged. This lowers the chance of injury and increases overall stability.

Furthermore, functional training can be customized to match each person's unique demands according to their age, fitness level, and objectives. While athletes may concentrate more on activities that increase power and agility for their particular activity, older folks may benefit from functional exercises that enhance balance and coordination to lower the risk of falls.

Finally, functional training is a very successful strategy for raising functional fitness and general quality of life. Functional training includes movement patterns, multi-joint exercises, core stability, and customized programming to help people of all ages and fitness levels become more confident and comfortable performing daily tasks. Functional training offers a comprehensive strategy that can help you reach your goals and lead a healthier, more active life, whether your focus is on improving your strength, flexibility, balance, or general fitness.

7.2 - ADVANTAGES FOR ENHANCING ROUTINE TASKS

Numerous advantages are provided by functional training for enhancing daily tasks and general quality of life. Improved strength and endurance are two main advantages; these are necessary for carrying out activities like pushing, lifting, and carrying things. You can make these chores easier and lower your risk of strain or injury by using functional training to improve the muscles involved in these activities.

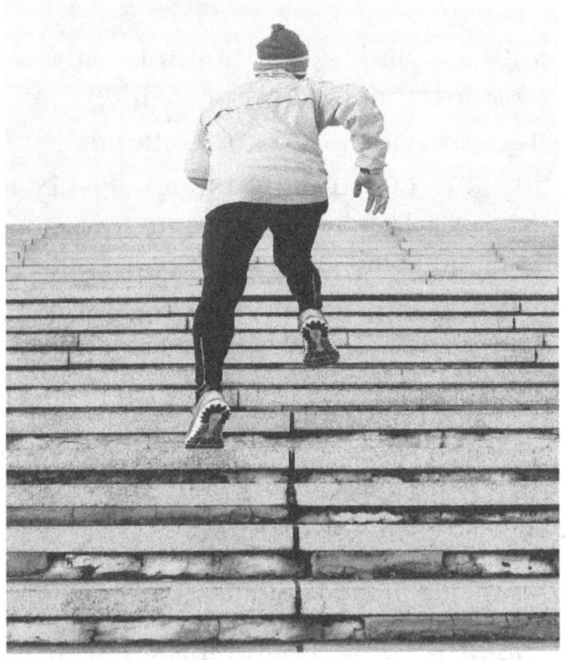

Enhancing balance and stability is another benefit of functional exercise. These abilities are essential for tasks like walking, climbing stairs, and getting up from a seated position. You can enhance your ability to execute balance and stability exercises safely and confidently by including exercises like single-leg stands or balancing board exercises.

Functional exercise can also aid in enhancing range of motion and flexibility, both of which are critical for tasks requiring reaching, twisting, or bending. Stretching exercises can help you become more flexible and lower your chance of getting hurt while doing everyday tasks.

Additionally, functional training aids in posture correction, which is necessary to preserve the spine's natural alignment and lower the likelihood of shoulder, neck, and back problems. You can maintain proper posture all day long with the support of functional training, which strengthens the core muscles and enhances body awareness.

Increased agility and coordination are two other advantages of functional training, which are critical for tasks requiring fast, accurate movements. Exercises that test your agility and coordination, such agility ladder drills or cone drills, will help you become more proficient at completing these tasks quickly and accurately.

Additionally, functional training might enhance wellbeing and mental health. In general, exercise is known to release endorphins, which are feel-good and stress-relieving chemicals in the brain. You can get these advantages for your mental health and physical fitness by adding functional exercise into your routine.

Last but not least, functional training provides a comprehensive strategy for raising everyday functioning and general quality of life. Functional training can help you live a better, more active lifestyle by concentrating on strength, balance, flexibility, coordination, and mental health. It can also help you accomplish daily tasks more confidently and efficiently.

7.3 - EXAMPLES OF FUNCTIONAL EXERCISES

Functional exercises work a variety of muscle groups and movement patterns to enhance the body's capacity to carry out daily tasks more effectively and securely. Strength, balance, flexibility, and coordination can all be enhanced with these exercises, which simulate actions found in daily life. Here are a few illustrations of practical exercises:

1. Squats: Squats are a basic functional exercise that work the quadriceps, hamstrings, and glutes, among other lower body muscles. This exercise is a fantastic method to increase hip and leg flexibility and power since it replicates the motion of sitting and standing up.

2. Lunges: Another great functional exercise that works the lower body muscles as well as the core and stabilizing muscles is the lunge. This exercise can aid with balance, coordination, and strengthening in the legs and hips since it replicates the motion of walking.

3. Kettlebell Swings : This dynamic functional fitness focuses on the muscles of the posterior chain, which includes the lower back, glutes, and hamstrings. To work your core and lower body muscles, swing a kettlebell between your legs and up to shoulder height.

4. Deadlifts : A compound exercise, deadlifts work the muscles in the core, hamstrings, glutes, and lower back. This exercise can assist increase lower body and back strength and stability by simulating the motion of lifting large things off the ground.

5. Push-ups: A traditional functional exercise, push-ups work the muscles in the arms, shoulders, core, and chest. This exercise can assist in increasing upper body strength and stability since it simulates lifting yourself up off the ground.

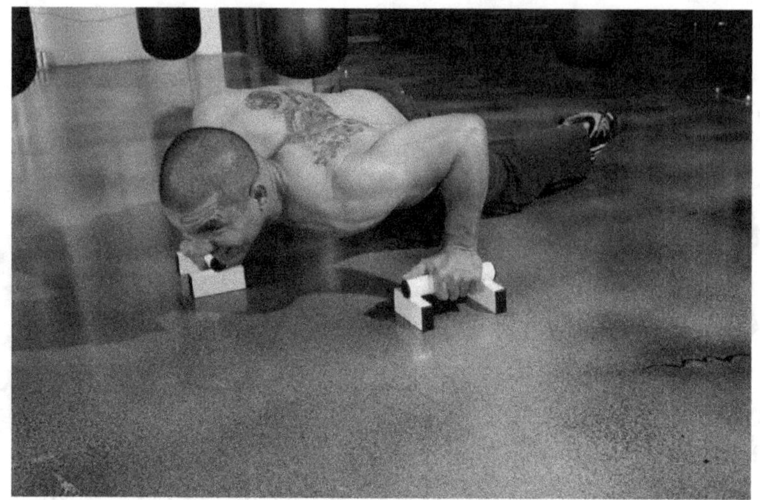

6. Pull-ups: Another excellent and effective functional exercise, pull-ups work the arms, core, shoulders, and back muscles. This exercise can assist in increasing upper body strength and stability since it simulates the motion of lifting oneself up.

7. Planks: A static functional exercise, planks work the arms, shoulders, and core muscles. This exercise can help strengthen and stabilize the core by having the person sustain a push-up position while keeping their body straight.

8. Medicine Ball tosses: A dynamic functional workout, medicine ball tosses work the arms, shoulders, and core muscles. To strengthen the core and upper body muscles, try throwing a medicine ball to a partner or against a wall.

9. Step-ups: Step-ups engage the muscles in the legs, hips, and core. They are a functional workout. This exercise can assist in increasing leg strength and stability since it simulates the motion of climbing stairs.

10. Balance Exercises : Balance exercises, including utilizing a balancing board or standing on one leg, can assist increase stability and balance, both of which are necessary for daily tasks. These activities can lower the chance of falling and enhance proprioception.

Including these functional workouts in your program will help you become more fit overall and make performing daily tasks safer and easier. As you get more comfortable, start with bodyweight exercises and progressively up the complexity and intensity. Always employ appropriate form and technique to minimize risks of injury and to get the most out of each of the exercises.

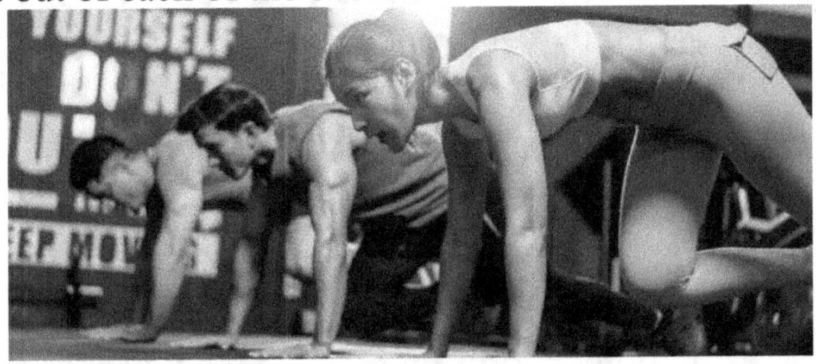

7.4 - HOW TO EMBRACE FUNCTIONAL TRAINING IN YOUR EXERCISE REGIMEN

Embracing functional training in your fitness regimen will help you become more functionally fit overall and make performing daily tasks safer and easier. The following advice can help you include functional training in your daily routine:

1. Evaluate Your Objectives: Prior to adding functional training to your regimen, evaluate your objectives and pinpoint areas that need work. Choose the everyday tasks you wish to enhance and modify your functional training workouts accordingly.

2. Start cautiously : To prevent overdoing it and getting hurt, begin functional training cautiously if you're new to it. Start with simple exercises like planks, lunges, and squats, and as you get more comfortable, progressively up the difficulty and intensity.

3. Pay Attention to Movement Patterns : During functional exercises, pay more attention to movement patterns than to discrete muscle actions. This entails using a variety of joints and muscle groups to simulate movements found in real life.

4. Include Variety : Include a range of functional activities in your regimen to guarantee a well-rounded workout. Exercises that focus on various muscle groups and movement patterns, such medicine ball tosses, kettlebell swings, squats, and lunges, can fall under this category.

5. Use Functional Equipmen t: To add variation and difficulty to your practice, think about utilizing functional equipment like medicine balls, balancing boards, kettlebells, and resistance bands. Enhancing strength, balance, and coordination can be facilitated by these techniques.

6. Combine with Other Exercises: Strength training, flexibility training, and cardiovascular exercise can all be included in a more comprehensive fitness regimen that incorporates functional training. Combining functional exercises with other exercise kinds will help you work out in a variety of ways.

7. Advance Gradually : As you get more accustomed to functional training, progressively up the level of difficulty and intensity in your exercises. This can involve introducing new variants, extending the time spent performing exercises, or boosting resistance.

8. Listen to Your Body: During and after functional training exercises, pay attention to how your body feels. Should you feel any pain or discomfort, cease the workout right once and seek medical advice if needed.

9. Be Consistent: When adding functional training to your regimen, consistency is essential, just like with any other type of exercise. For increases in functional fitness, try to engage in functional activities two or three times a week.

10. Monitor Your Progress : Keep a journal of your workouts and note any gains you make in terms of coordination, strength, and balance. Honor your accomplishments and utilize failures as teaching moments to modify your program as necessary.

By including these functional training into your fitness regimen, you may increase your functional fitness level overall and make performing daily tasks safer and easier. To get the best results, start out gently, concentrate on movement patterns, add diversity, use functional equipment, combine with other workouts, proceed gradually, pay attention to your body, be consistent, and monitor your progress.

8.0 INTERVAL TRAINING FOR EFFECTIVE WORKOUTS

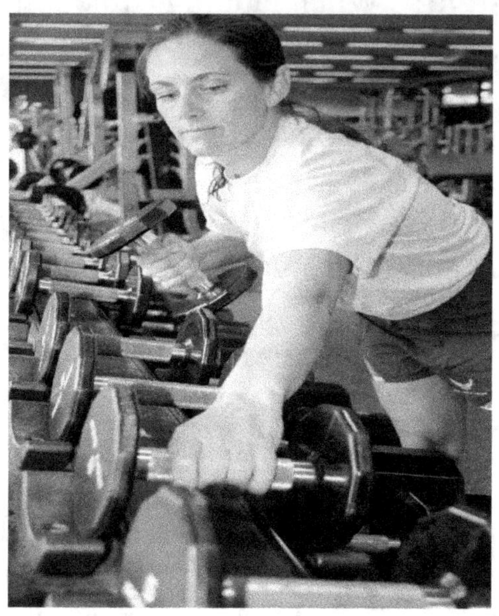

8.1 INTERVAL TRAINING

An exercise regimen known as interval training alternates between high-intensity and low-intensity intervals, or rest intervals. By pushing your body to its limits during the high-intensity intervals and allowing for recuperation during the lower-intensity intervals, interval training aims to maximize the effectiveness of your workout.

The idea of "interval," which refers to the precise amount of time for each workout phase, is the fundamental idea of interval training. You put up your greatest effort during the high-intensity periods, raising your respiration and heart rates to their maximum points. This increases fat and calorie burning while also enhancing cardiovascular fitness and endurance.

Conversely, you give your body time to heal and get ready for the subsequent high-intensity phase during the lower-intensity intervals, also known as rest periods. You can sustain intensity throughout the entire workout by avoiding exhaustion and overexertion during this recovery phase.

Various exercises, including bodyweight exercises, cycling, swimming, and running, can be incorporated into interval training. For instance, in a running session, you might alternate between sprinting and strolling, and in a cycling training, between high- and low-resistance riding.

The effectiveness of interval training is one of its key advantages. Compared to steady-state cardio, interval training can offer a more efficient workout in less time since it varies between high- and low-intensity periods. Because of this, it's a fantastic choice for those who have hectic schedules yet still want to get in a good workout.

The rate of metabolism can also be boosted by interval training. Your body must work harder and burn more calories during and after the workout due to the high-intensity intervals, which raises your metabolic rate. Even when you're not exercising, this can help you burn extra calories throughout the day.

Interval training also has the potential to increase both anaerobic and aerobic fitness. The high-intensity intervals increase your body's capability for aerobic exercise, or how well it uses oxygen. Your body's ability to do brief, powerful bursts of activity without oxygen is known as your anaerobic capacity, and it is improved by the low-intensity intervals or rest periods.

In conclusion, interval training is a very successful form of exercise that can raise metabolism, burn calories, enhance cardiovascular fitness, and enhance both anaerobic and aerobic fitness. Including interval training in your exercise regimen can help you reach your fitness objectives faster and more successfully.

8.2 - ADVANTAGES FOR INCREASING HEART HEALTH AND BURNING FAT

There are many advantages to interval training for increasing heart health and burning calories. Its capacity to increase cardiovascular fitness faster than steady-state cardio exercise is one of its main advantages. Interval training tests your cardiovascular system by alternating between high- and low-intensity intervals, which can enhance your heart health and general endurance.

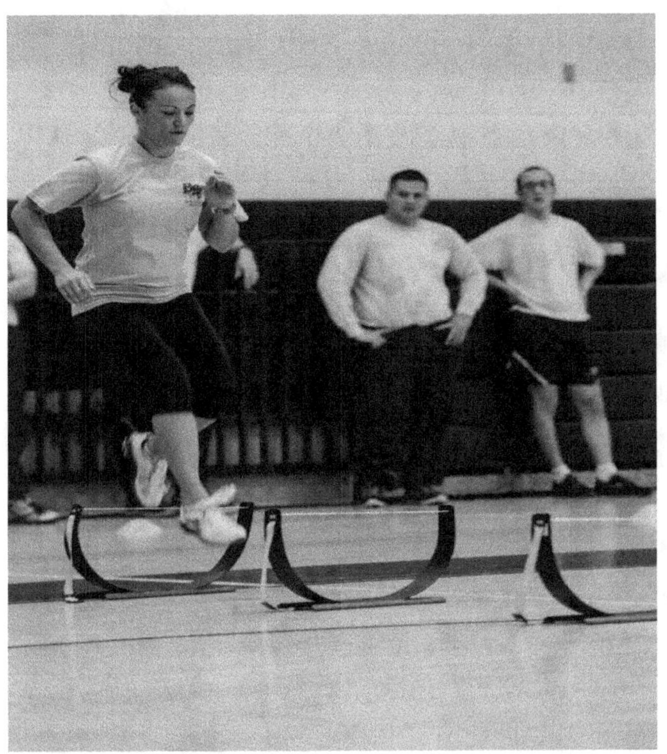

Your heart rate rises dramatically during the high-intensity intervals, which makes your heart work harder to pump blood and oxygen to your muscles. This promotes increased cardiac muscle strength and efficiency, which enhances general cardiovascular fitness. This may eventually result in improved blood pressure, a decreased risk of cardiovascular disease, and a lower resting heart rate.

Another efficient method for burning calories and decreasing weight is interval exercise. Your body is pushed to its maximum capacity during the high-intensity intervals, which increases calorie burn during and after the workout. This phenomenon, which occurs even after you've completed exercising, is called the "afterburn effect" or excess post-exercise oxygen consumption, or

EPOC. You can burn more calories with this compared to the residual state cardio.

Interval training can also help you burn more calories. The growth hormone produced by the high-intensity interval training boosts metabolism and aids in fat burning. This can help you maintain a healthy weight and body composition by increasing the amount of calories you burn even when you're not exercising.

Moreover, interval training helps control blood sugar levels and enhance insulin sensitivity. Your muscles' glycogen stores are depleted during the high-intensity intervals, which enhances your body's capacity to use insulin and control blood sugar. Those who have diabetes or insulin resistance may benefit most from this.

Interval training can also help you become more fit overall and perform better in other pursuits. You may increase your speed, power, and endurance with high-intensity interval training, which can help you perform better in sports and other physical activities.

Ultimately, interval training is a very successful exercise technique for increasing cardiovascular fitness, burning calories, and reaching weight loss objectives. You may take advantage of interval training's numerous advantages and lead a more active, healthy lifestyle by including it into your exercise regimen.

8.3 -EXAMPLES OF EXERCISES INCLUDING INTERVAL TRAINING (E.G., HIIT, TABATA)

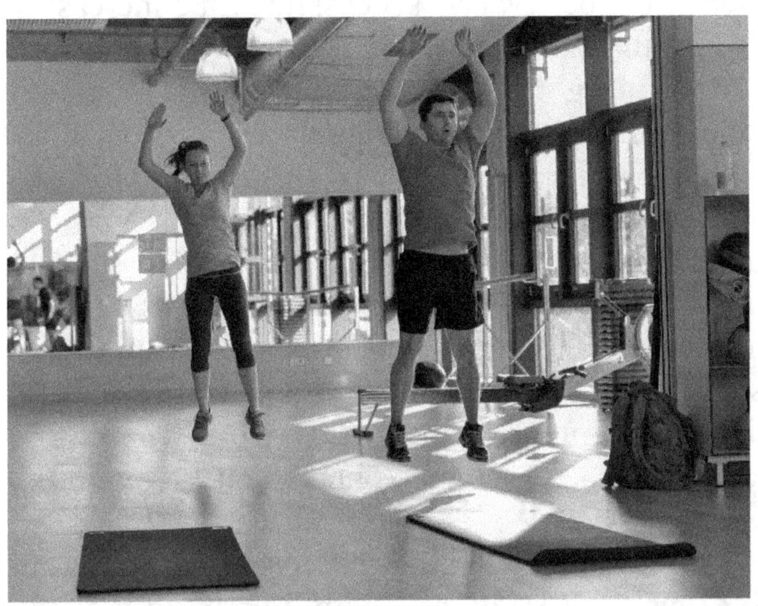

There are several ways to conduct interval training, but two of the most well-liked techniques are Tabata and High-Intensity Interval Training (HIIT). These exercises are well renowned for their ability to raise metabolism, burn calories, and improve cardiovascular fitness. These are a few samples of interval training exercises:

1. High-Intensity Interval Training (HIIT): HIIT alternates brief bursts of high-intensity exercise with rest intervals or lower-intensity workouts. For instance, you may sprint for thirty seconds, take a thirty-second break, and then repeat the process multiple times. You can add a range of exercises to your HIIT routines, like burpees, running, cycling, jumping jacks, and mountain climbers.

2. Tabata : Tabata is a type of high-intensity interval training (HIIT) that consists of eight rounds, or four minutes, of 20 seconds of extremely intense exercise followed by 10 seconds of relaxation. Dr. Izumi Tabata, a scientist from Japan, created this method, which has been demonstrated to be very successful in increasing cardiovascular fitness and burning calories.

3. Interval Running : This type of running alternates sprinting and walking or jogging intervals. For instance, you could run for one minute, then jog or walk for two minutes, and so on for a number of repetitions. You can perform this outside, on a treadmill, or on a track.

4. Interval Cycling : This technique entails switching between intervals of high and low resistance or high and low intensity. For instance, you may bike for one minute at a high resistance or intensity, then recover for two minutes at a reduced resistance or intensity, and so on for a number of rounds.

5. Circuit Training : This type of exercise is carrying out a sequence of tasks, or "stations," with little to no break in between. Every station concentrates on a distinct muscular group or gait. You may, for instance, execute a circuit of bodyweight exercises like planks, squats, lunges, and push-ups, holding each pose for 30 to 60 seconds before switching to the next station.

6. Pyramid Intervals : Pyramid intervals entail progressively raising and lowering the intervals' duration or intensity. For instance, you may begin with a sprint of 30 seconds, then rest for 30 seconds, then raise to a 45-second sprint, then rest for 45 seconds, and so on, until you return to a 30-second sprint.

7. Fartlek Training : Fartlek, which translates to "speed play" from Swedish, is an interval training style in which you change up the pace and intensity of your exercises. This can be achieved by sprinting or cycling for a little amount of time or distance, then relaxing for a while.

These are only a few instances of interval training exercises; you can attempt a lot of other versions and combinations. It's important to push yourself during the high-intensity intervals and give yourself enough time to recover during lower-intensity intervals or rest. A difficult but effective exercise technique that can help you reach your fitness objectives and raise your level of fitness is interval training.

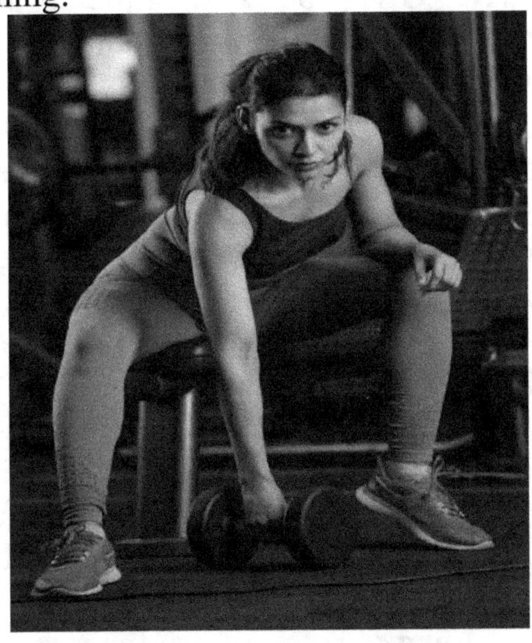

8.4 - HOW TO SECURELY CARRY OUT INTERVAL TRAINING

A great exercise technique for raising metabolism, burning calories, and enhancing cardiovascular fitness is interval training. To prevent injury and optimize the effects of your exercise, interval training must be done safely. The following advice can help you practice interval training safely:

1. Get warmed up Correctly : Warming up your muscles and cardiovascular system before beginning an interval training session is crucial to preparing them for the strenuous exertion that lies ahead. To improve flexibility and blood flow, try some light cardio, dynamic stretches, and mobility drills.

2. Start Slowly: Give your body time to adjust to the intensity of interval training if you're new to it. As you get more comfortable, progressively increase the duration and intensity. Start with shorter intervals and lower intensities.

3. Listen to Your Body: Throughout the exercise, be aware of how your body is feeling. Stop the activity right away and take some time to relax if you feel any pain, lightheadedness, or discomfort. It is crucial to pay attention to your body's cues and modify the amount of time or intensity of your required intervals.

4. Stay Hydrated: Drink enough water when doing interval training, especially if you're doing intense workouts that make you perspire a lot. To stay hydrated and avoid dehydration before and after your workout, drink water.

5. Use Correct Form : To minimize the risk of injury and to get the most out of your workout, use correct form during all exercises. This entails utilizing controlled motions, maintaining a straight back, and using your core.

6. Gradually raise Intensity : To keep your body challenged as you get more accustomed to interval training, progressively raise the intensity of your intervals.

By doing this, you can gradually raise your level of fitness and avoid hitting plateaus.

7. Provide Enough Rest Periods : Your body needs enough time to recuperate and restore energy reserves between sessions. By doing this, you can lessen your risk of injury from overtraining and exhaustion.

8. Cool Down Correctly : To aid in your body's recovery after an interval training session, it's critical to cool down correctly. To help with muscle discomfort and relaxation, this can involve deep breathing exercises, static stretches, and light aerobics.

9. Listen to Your Body: Observe your body's sensations both during and following an exercise. Stop the activity right away and take some time to relax if you feel any pain, lightheadedness, or discomfort. It's critical to pay attention to your body's signals and modify the length or intensity of your intervals as necessary.

10. Maintain Consistency : When it comes to interval training, consistency is essential, just like it is with any type of exercise. For optimal results, try to routinely incorporate interval training into your exercise regimen.

You can safely engage in interval training and reap its many benefits for enhancing cardiovascular fitness, burning calories, and speeding up metabolism by using these pointers. To safely and successfully reach your fitness goals, always remember to start out cautiously, pay attention to your body, and maintain consistency.

9.0 CROSS-TRAINING FOR OVERALL FITNESS

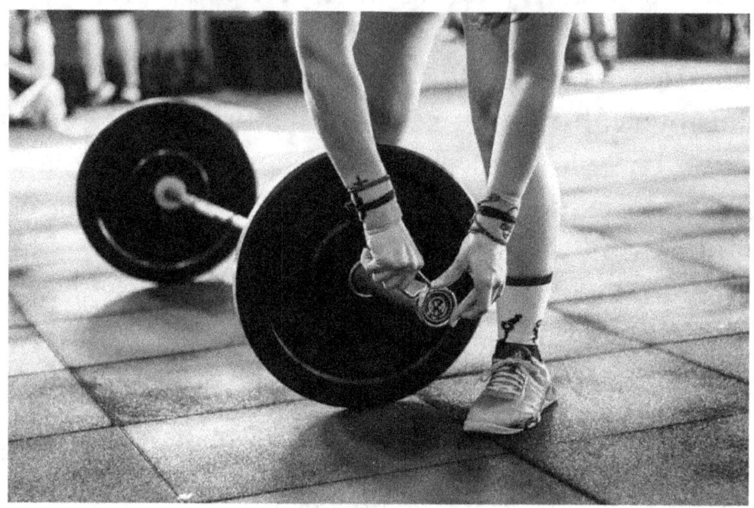

9.1 CROSS-TRAINING OVERVIEW

In order to increase overall fitness and avoid boredom or overuse problems, cross-training is a fitness technique that entails participating in a range of various exercises or activities. The premise behind cross-training is that you can target multiple muscle groups, increase cardiovascular fitness, and improve your overall performance in sports or other physical activities by including a variety of exercises into your program.

By keeping your workouts new and entertaining, cross-training helps minimize boredom, which is one of its main advantages. Running, cycling, swimming, strength training, and yoga are just a few of the activities you can mix up to keep yourself engaged and out of a fitness rut.

Preventing overuse injuries is an additional benefit of cross-training. Repetitive usage of the same kind of exercise or activity raises the risk of overuse injuries like stress fractures or tendinitis. You may lessen the chance of injury and give your muscles and joints a rest from repetitive motions by mixing up your routine with different exercises.

By concentrating on various muscular groups and energy systems, cross-training also aids in enhancing general fitness. Running, for instance, focuses more on the lower body muscles and cardiovascular system, whereas swimming trains the core and upper body muscles. Running and swimming together will help you reach a more comprehensive and well-balanced level of fitness.

Cross-training can also aid in enhancing athletic or other physical activity performance. Exercises that closely resemble the motions and requirements of your sport or activity might help you advance particular abilities and raise your game overall. A basketball player could utilize plyometrics and agility drills to increase speed and agility on the court, while a runner might employ strength training routines that focus on the leg muscles used in running.

In summary, cross-training is a very successful fitness strategy that can assist increase general fitness, guard against boredom and overuse issues, and improve athletic or other physical activity performance. Your program can help you reach a balanced level of fitness and get the many advantages of cross-training by including a variety of exercises.

9.2 - ADVANTAGES FOR AVOIDING FATIGUE AND OVERUSE INJURIES

The avoidance of overuse injuries and boredom are two important advantages of cross-training. Let's examine these advantages in more detail:

Preventing Boredom : Remaining consistent with a fitness regimen might be difficult because of boredom. Regularly performing the same workouts might cause monotony, which can make it challenging to maintain motivation. Cross-training adds diversity to your workouts, which helps keep you from getting bored. You may make your workouts exciting and engaging by mixing together different exercise forms, such as swimming, cycling, running, and strength training. This type can help you get greater results by stimulating your mind and forcing your body to work in novel ways.

Additionally, cross-training enables you to experiment with various activities to determine which ones you enjoy the most. This can assist in changing the perception of exercise from a chore to a pleasurable activity you do every day. Cross-training gives countless opportunities to keep your workouts interesting and pleasurable, whether you're hitting the pool for a swim, the trails for a run, or the gym for a strength training session.

Preventing Overuse Injuries: Repetitive exercisers such as athletes and fitness enthusiasts frequently suffer from overuse injuries. When the same muscles, tendons, and joints are repeatedly stressed without having adequate time to heal, these injuries happen. Strains in the muscles, stress fractures, and tendonitis are common overuse injuries.

By allowing you to switch up the muscles you utilize and the types of activities you do, cross-training helps prevent overuse problems. You can lessen the pressure on any one muscle group or joint by combining cardiovascular activities, strength training, and flexibility training. In addition to preventing overuse injuries, this enhances joint stability and total muscle balance.

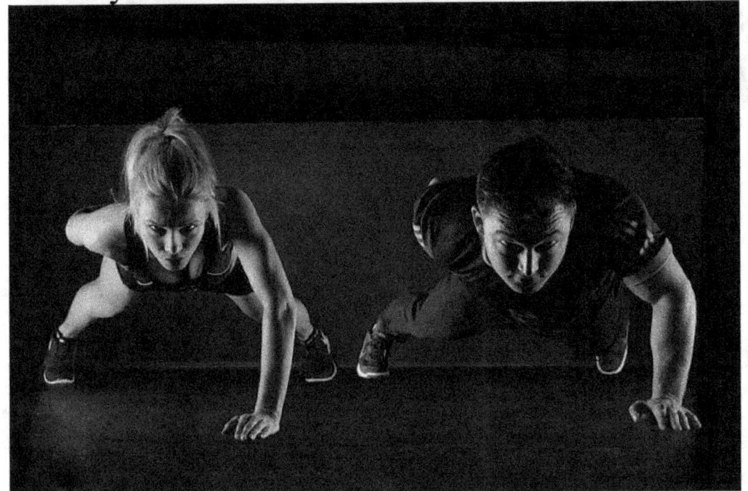

Cross-training can also assist in locating and correcting muscular imbalances that may be a factor in overuse problems. For instance, adding upper body strength training activities can help balance out your muscle development and minimize your chance of injury if you're a runner who predominantly uses your lower body muscles.

Moreover, cross-training is a useful tactic to avoid fatigue and overuse issues. You may lower your risk of overuse injuries and maintain an engaging and challenging fitness regimen by mixing up your routine and the activities you perform. Cross-training has a number of advantages that can help you safely and successfully reach your fitness objectives, regardless of your level of experience as an athlete or where you are in your fitness journey.

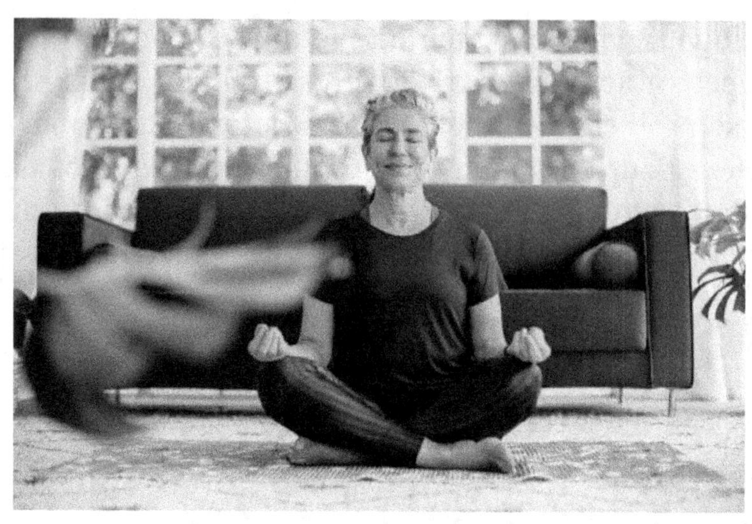

9.3 - DIFFERENT KINDS OF CROSS-TRAINING EXERCISES

To reach a balanced level of fitness, cross-train by including a range of activities into your exercise regimen. These are a few instances of cross-training exercises:

1. Swimming: Stretching the entire body, swimming is an excellent low-impact workout. Strength, flexibility, and cardiovascular fitness are all enhanced by it. Those with joint problems or injuries can benefit most from swimming.

2. Cycling : Riding a stationary bike indoors or outdoors is another low-impact workout option. It enhances endurance, cardiovascular fitness, and leg strength. Cycling is a fantastic choice for anyone seeking a productive yet low-impact exercise.

3. Strength Training: To increase muscle endurance and strength, strength trainers use weights or resistance bands. It can enhance bone density, muscular tone, and general strength. Exercises for strength training can include lunges, push-ups, dumbbell curls, and squats.

4. Yoga : Yoga is a mind-body discipline which includes breathing techniques, physical postures, and meditation. Strength, balance, flexibility, and relaxation are all enhanced by it. Yoga can help prevent injuries and is a terrific addition to other forms of fitness.

5. Pilates: Pilates is an exercise style that targets body awareness, flexibility, and strengthening of the core muscles. It can aid with balance, coordination, and posture. Pilates is frequently performed on a mat or with specific apparatus like a reformer.

6. Dance: Cardiovascular fitness, coordination, and flexibility can all be enhanced via dancing, an enjoyable and energizing type of exercise. There are numerous dancing forms, including salsa, ballet, and hip-hop, each with certain advantages of its own.

7. High-Intensity Interval Training, or HIIT , is a type of exercise that alternates short bursts of vigorous activity with rest intervals or lower-intensity workouts. It can raise metabolism, burn calories, and enhance cardiovascular fitness.

8. Sports : Playing sports like volleyball, basketball, tennis, or soccer can be an enjoyable and difficult kind of exercise. Agility, coordination, cardiovascular fitness, and teamwork are all enhanced by sports.

9. Hiking: Getting outside and taking in the scenery while getting a decent workout is possible through hiking. It enhances endurance, leg strength, and cardiovascular fitness.

10. Rowing: Rowing is a fantastic full-body exercise that enhances strength, endurance, and cardiovascular fitness. You can do it on the water or with a rowing machine.

These are but a handful of types of cross-training exercises. The secret to creating a well-rounded exercise regimen is to find enjoyable activities that push your body in new ways.

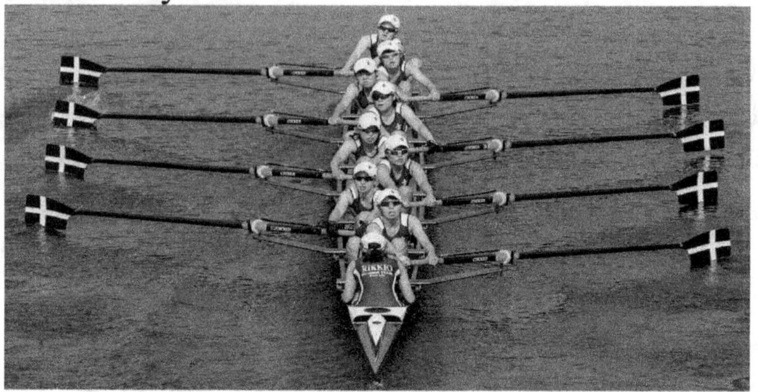

9.4 HOW TO DRAFT A PLAN FOR CROSS-TRAINING

To attain a well-rounded and efficient exercise program, cross-training is adding a variety of activities to your fitness regimen. The steps to establishing a cross-training strategy are as follows:

1. Establish Your Goals : It's critical to ascertain your fitness objectives prior to devising a cross-training regimen. Your cross-training strategy will be guided by your goals, whether they are to increase general fitness, gain strength, lose weight, or improve cardiovascular fitness.

2. Pick Your Exercises: Opt for a range of exercises that focus on several facets of health, including strength, flexibility, balance, and cardiovascular fitness. Exercises like swimming, cycling, weight training, yoga, Pilates, and dance are a few examples.

3. Make a Schedule: Choose how frequently you will engage in cross-training each week and how you will allocate your time. For instance, you may schedule three to five cross-training sessions per week, each lasting between thirty and sixty minutes.

4. Mix It Up : To keep your workouts engaging and difficult, include a variety of activities in your schedule. For instance, you may spend the week switching between weight training, cycling, and swimming.

5. Progress Gradually : As your fitness level rises, start out cautiously and progressively increase the volume, duration, and frequency of your workouts. This will guarantee continuous development toward your goals and help prevent injuries.

6. Listen to Your Body: Keep an eye on how your body reacts to various exercises and modify your strategy as necessary. In the event that you feel pain or discomfort, cease the activity and seek medical advice.

7. Allocate Rest Days: To help your body recuperate and avoid overtraining, incorporate rest days into your cross-training regimen. Rest days are essential to reaching your fitness objectives and should be treated with the same importance as workout days.

8. Remain Consistent : To get the best results, try your hardest to adhere to your cross-training schedule. Maintaining a healthy lifestyle and reaching your fitness objectives require consistency.

9. Monitor Your Progress : Record the exercises you perform, their duration, and their intensity. This will assist you in tracking your development and modifying your plan as necessary.

10. Remain Motivated: Discover strategies to maintain your enthusiasm for your exercises. Whether it's through goal-setting, experimenting, or working out with friends, maintaining your motivation can help you follow through on your cross-training regimen and meet your fitness objectives.

These steps will help you design a cross-training program that meets your fitness objectives and assists you in completing a well-rounded and efficient exercise regimen.

10.0 MUSCLE REPAIR AND RECOVERY

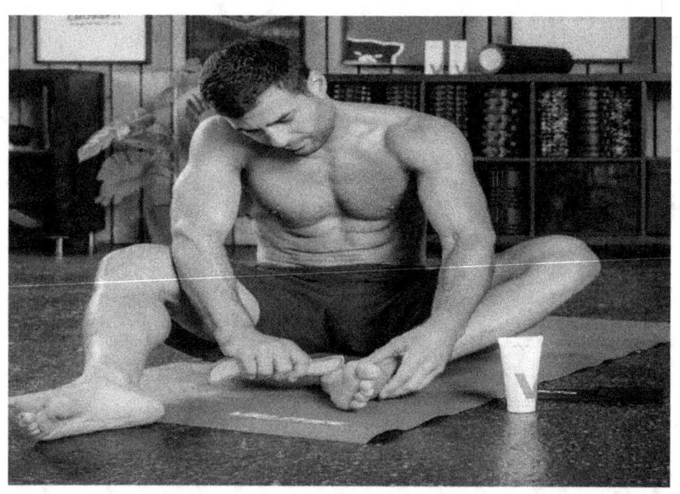

10.1 - THE IMPACT OF REST AND RECOVERY IN A FITNESS PROGRAM

The cornerstones of every successful fitness regimen are rest and recuperation. They are essential for the growth, repair, and general improvement of muscle performance.

Muscles experience tension and microscopic rips when exercising, particularly during high-intensity sessions. These muscles can heal and get stronger during times of rest and recuperation. Muscles may not have the time to heal completely without adequate rest, which could result in overtraining and a higher risk of injury.

When the body is not given enough time to rest and recuperate between sessions, overtraining is a prevalent problem. This may lead to exhaustion, a decline in performance, and an increased risk of injury. The body may fully recover from overtraining when there is adequate rest.

Getting enough sleep and recovering from injuries also helps you perform better. Muscles that have had enough sleep can function at their best, improving strength, endurance, and general fitness. Rest also promotes mental renewal, which lowers stress and enhances motivation and focus for ensuing workouts.

The recovery process and rest are essential for preventing injuries. Overtraining raises the risk of injury by causing weariness, decreased coordination, and muscular imbalances. Getting enough sleep promotes general physical health and helps avert these problems.

Rest intervals are also necessary to maintain the immune system. Excessive physical activity has the potential to momentarily impair immunity, increasing susceptibility to disease. Rest lowers the risk of disease and infection by enabling the immune system to repair and perform at its best.

Another essential component of rest and recuperation is hormone control. Getting enough sleep helps the body produce growth hormone, which is essential for building and repairing muscles. Hormone balance plays a role in general fitness and health.

Last but not least, recovery and rest encourage improved sleep, which is essential for general health and wellbeing. While overtraining might interfere with sleep patterns, exercise can enhance the quality of sleep. Better sleep is made possible by rest times, which promote healing and general wellness.

In summary, relaxation and recuperation are critical elements of an effective exercise regimen. They help build and repair muscles, guard against overtraining and injuries, enhance performance, strengthen the immune system, balance hormones, and encourage sound sleep. The secret to safely and successfully reaching your fitness objectives is incorporating enough rest and recovery intervals into your exercise routine.

10.2 THE ADVANTAGES OF RELAXATION FOR MUSCLE GROWTH AND HEALING

Muscle growth and repair depend on rest. Physical activity causes small tears in your muscle fibers, particularly in strength training and resistance workouts. Your muscles get stronger and more resilient as a result of your body repairing these tears during rest periods. The following are the main advantages of rest for muscle growth and repair:

1. Muscle Repair: Your muscles can heal from the harm that comes from exercise when you are at rest. Muscle growth and strength are produced as a result of this repair process, which creates new muscle protein strands to replace damaged ones.

2. Muscle Growth : Muscle hypertrophy, or the growth of muscles, depends on rest. Your body enlarges muscle fibers when you're at rest in order to prepare them for the demands of your exercise. Strengthening and gaining muscle mass require this process.

3. Refueling of Energy Stores : During sleep, your body can restock on energy reserves like glycogen, which serves as your muscles' main energy source when you exercise. Your muscles will have adequate energy for maximum performance and recovery if you get enough sleep.

4. Hormone Regulation : Hormones essential for muscle growth and repair, such as testosterone and growth hormone (GH), are released during rest. Deep sleep causes a greater release of these hormones, underscoring the significance of getting enough sleep for effective muscle health.

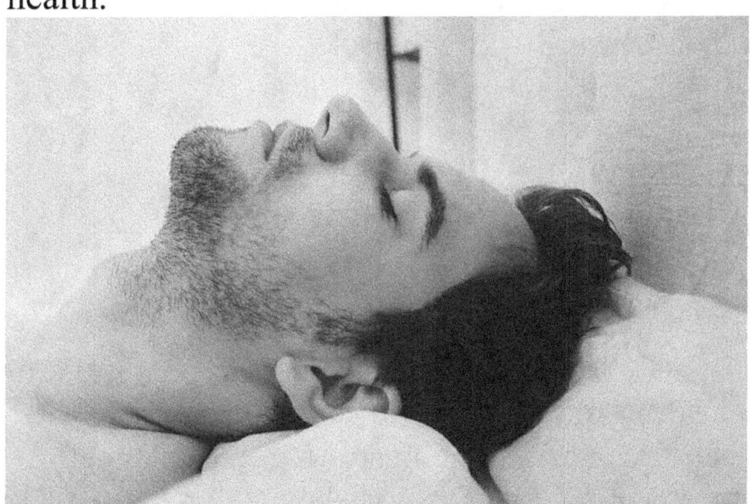

5. Preventing Overtraining : Overtraining is a condition marked by weariness, diminished performance, and an elevated risk of injury. Rest helps avoid overtraining. When the body is not given adequate time to recuperate between sessions, overtraining takes place. Resting enough facilitates complete recuperation and lowers the chance of overtraining.

6. Inflammation Reduction : Vigorous exercise can cause muscle inflammation, which is a normal aspect of the healing process. Rest aids in reducing inflammation, which promotes quicker healing and decreased discomfort in the muscles.

7. Optimal Performance : To function at your best, you must get enough sleep. Your ability to lift large weights, run quicker, and perform better overall as an athlete is enhanced by well-rested muscles.

In summary, sleep is essential for muscle growth and repair. It enables your muscles to heal injuries, restore stored energy, balance hormones, stop overtraining, lessen inflammation, and function at their best. Getting enough sleep is a crucial part of any workout regimen if you want to safely and successfully grow muscle.

10.3 - TECHNIQUES FOR FITTING RELAXATION AND REPAIR INTO A TRAINING ROUTINE

A plan that balances work and relaxation is necessary to keep up a healthy and productive exercise regimen. The following tactics can assist you in striking this balance:

1. Listen to Your Body: Observe how your body feels both during and following exercise. It can be an indication that you need more sleep if you feel tired or sore. Conversely, however,if you feel energized and ready to go, you may be ready to tackle a more intense workout.

2. Plan Your exercises : Make sure you have a good balance between rest and intensity by planning your exercises ahead of time. Plan rest days into your routine to give yourself time to recover in between workouts.

3. Switch Between tough and Lighter Days: Switch between hard training sessions and more relaxed, recuperation-oriented sessions. This can lessen the chance of injury and assist avoid overtraining.

4. Employ a Training Plan: Adhere to a regimented training plan that incorporates periodization, which is gradually increasing the volume and intensity of your workouts. In addition to preventing burnout, this can enhance performance.

5. Incorporate Active Recovery : Schedule days for low-intensity exercises like yoga, stretching, or walking as part of your active recovery regimen. In order to improve blood flow to the muscles and lessen stiffness, active rehabilitation can be helpful.

6. Make Sleep a Priority: Make sure you get adequate sleep to promote muscle growth and repair. Aim for 7-9 hours of good sleep every night because it's necessary for healing and general well-being.

7. Drink Plenty of Water and Eat Well : Eating right and staying hydrated are essential for healing. To encourage muscle growth and repair, nourish your body with nutrient-rich foods and stay hydrated.

8. Pay Attention to Your Mind : Mental and physical exhaustion are equally significant. Feeling mentally exhausted could indicate that you need to take a break from tough workouts.

Think about adding mindfulness or meditation to your routine as ways to relieve stress.

9. Be Adaptable : Allow yourself to change your plans according to your emotional state. Do not hesitate to take an additional rest day if necessary. It is preferable to take it easy and heal rather than strain yourself and become hurt.

10. Track Your Progress : To ascertain whether you're striking the correct balance between work and relaxation, keep a log of your workouts and your overall well-being. To make sure you're receiving enough sleep to support your exercise objectives, make any necessary scheduling adjustments.

By including these tactics into your routine, you can get a well-rounded approach to fitness that encompasses both exercise and relaxation. Maintaining this balance is crucial for reaching long-term fitness objectives, enhancing performance, and avoiding injuries.

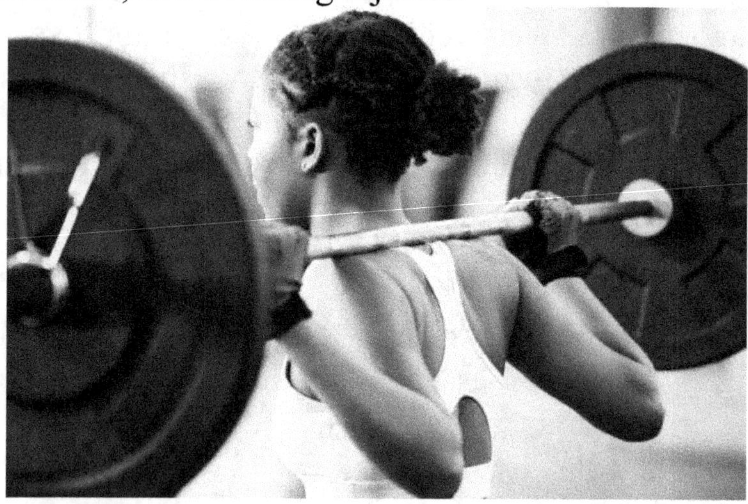

10.4- HOW TO PAY ATTENTION TO YOUR BODY AND STEER CLEAR OF EXCESSIVE EXERCISE

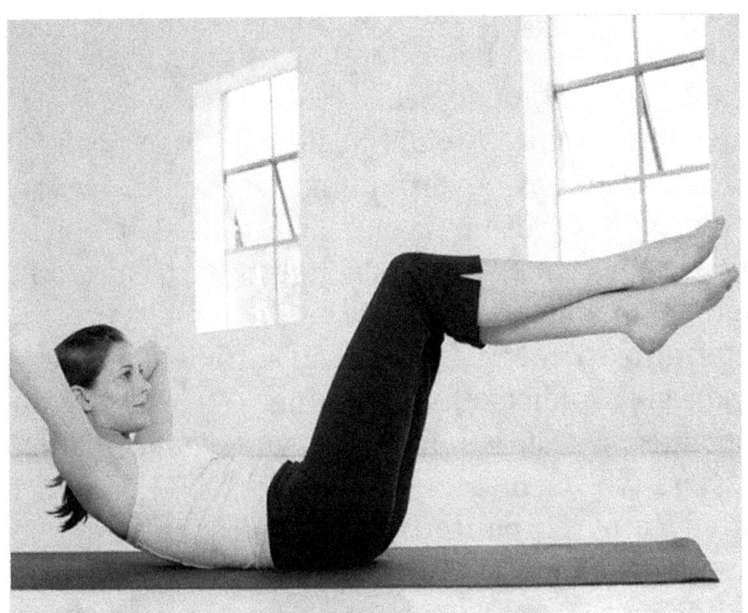

It's critical to pay attention to your body in order to prevent overtraining and preserve a balanced exercise regimen. To avoid overtraining, pay attention to your body in the following important ways:

1. Pay Attention to Fatigue : If you find yourself feeling worn out or exhausted all the time, you might be overtraining. Throughout the day, keep track of your energy levels and modify the intensity of your workouts accordingly.

2. Pay Attention to Muscle stiffness: Especially when attempting new exercises or stepping up the intensity, some stiffness in your muscles is natural after a workout.

On the other hand, chronic or severe soreness could indicate that you require additional sleep.

3. Keep an Eye Out for Performance Changes: Overtraining may be indicated if you observe an abrupt decline in performance, such as difficulty lifting weights that you would typically be able to lift or a slower pace during aerobic exercises. Pay attention to your body and allow yourself enough time to heal.

4. Examine Your Mood : Mental health and mood can be negatively impacted by overtraining. It could be an indication that you're pushing yourself too hard if you're feeling agitated, nervous, or melancholy. Step back and give rest and recuperation first priority.

5. Pay Attention to Sleep Habits : Insufficient or poor quality sleep may indicate overtraining. To assist with healing and muscle restoration, make sure you're getting adequate restorative sleep.

6. Evaluate Your Appetite : Your appetite may be impacted by overtraining. Your body may be under stress and in need of more rest if you're noticing fluctuations in your appetite, such as increased or decreased hunger.

7. Pay Attention to Pain: Although some soreness is typical with exercise, pain is not. It's crucial to halt and evaluate the situation if you're feeling intense or chronic discomfort during or after exercise. Exercise through pain might cause catastrophic harm if done incorrectly.

8. Recognize Your Tension Levels : Physical tension is something that exercise puts the body through. It's crucial to be aware of how much extra stress exercising puts on your body if you're already experiencing a lot of stress from other aspects of your life.

9. Take Rest Days : To help your body heal, schedule regular rest days into your schedule. In order to avoid overtraining, rest days are equally as crucial as workout days.

10. Modify Your Intensity: Don't be scared to change the volume or intensity of your workout if you're feeling exhausted or overtrained. Pay attention to your body and allow yourself to rest when necessary.

In summary, it is critical to pay attention to your body in order to prevent overtraining and preserve a balanced exercise regimen. Keep an eye out for symptoms of exhaustion, track soreness in your muscles, keep an eye out for changes in your performance, take into account your mood, evaluate your appetite, keep an eye on your sleep patterns, listen to pain, be aware of your stress levels, take days off, and modify your intensity as necessary. You may prevent overtraining and keep moving in the direction of your fitness objectives by paying attention to your body and making rest and recovery a priority.

11.0 NUTRITION AND HYDRATION

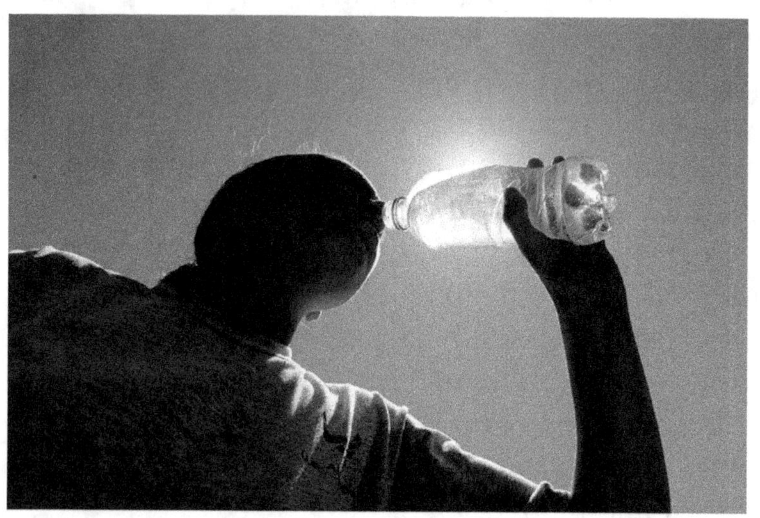

11.1 THE SIGNIFICANCE OF PROPER NUTRITION AND HYDRATION FOR EFFECTIVE EXERCISE

Hydration and a healthy diet are essential for doing an exercise program well. They give your body the nutrition and energy it needs to function at its peak. Here are some reasons why proper diet and hydration are crucial for effective exercise:

1. Energy Source : When you exercise, the energy required for your muscles to contract is obtained from food. The body uses carbohydrates as its main energy source, particularly while engaging in high-intensity activity. Consuming a diet high in carbohydrates guarantees that your muscles will have enough fuel to function at their best.

2. Muscle development and Repair: Both muscle development and repair depend on protein. Muscle fibers sustain tiny injury during exercising. After an exercise, consuming protein aids in the rebuilding of these fibers and the development of new muscle tissue, which eventually improves strength and endurance.

3. Hydration: Sustaining optimal performance requires adequate hydration. Water is necessary for carrying nutrients, lubricating joints, and controlling body temperature. Exhaustion, cramping, and poor performance can result from dehydration. To stay hydrated, it's critical to consume lots of liquids before, during, and following exercise.

4. Electrolyte Balance: Essential for proper muscle contraction and hydration are minerals including sodium, potassium, and magnesium. Sweating causes electrolyte loss during exercise. Maintaining muscle function and avoiding cramps is made possible by replenishing these electrolytes through a healthy diet and amount of water.

5. Nutrient Timing : Your ability to exercise might also be affected by when you eat. Prior to exercise, eating a well-balanced lunch or snack high in protein and carbs can aid avoid muscle breakdown and serve as a source of energy. In a similar vein, eating protein and carbohydrates after working out can help with muscle regeneration and recuperation.

6. Immune Function: The immune system may become momentarily compromised by exercise. Maintaining constant exercise performance is made possible by a proper diet, which includes getting enough vitamins and minerals. It also helps boost immune function and lowers the chance of illness or infection.

7. Mental Focus : During exercise, mental focus and concentration are influenced by nutrition. Consuming a diet rich in healthy fats, proteins, and carbohydrates gives your brain the nourishment it needs to function at its peak during physical activity.

8. General Health: Eating well and staying hydrated promote general health and wellbeing, both of which are necessary for long-term exercise performance. Maintaining good health and energy levels is facilitated by a diet rich in nutrients and balanced in a variety of foods.

In summary, proper diet and hydration are critical for optimal exercise performance. They give your body the vitality, nourishment, and moisture it needs to function at its peak. You may maximize your exercise performance and reach your fitness objectives by eating a balanced diet that includes a range of nutrient-dense meals and drinking plenty of water.

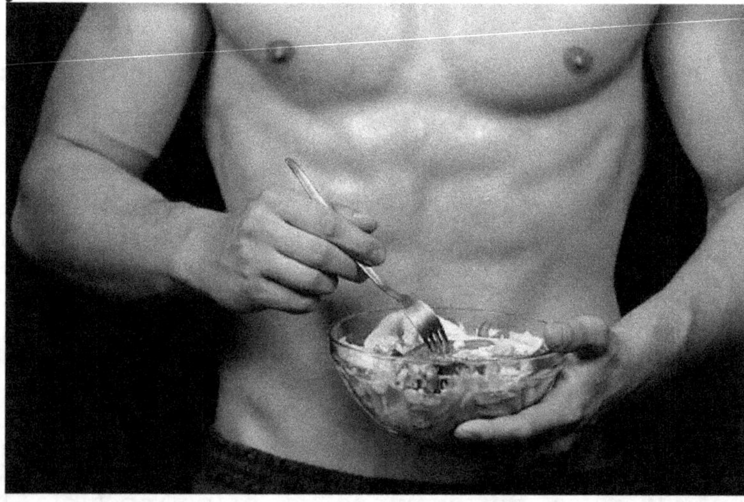

11.2 TIPS FOR PRE-EXERCISE NUTRITION

For your body to have the energy and nutrients it needs to function at its peak during exercise, pre-exercise nutrition is essential. The following pre-exercise dietary advice can help you maximize your workouts:

1. Consume a Balanced Meal: Two to three hours before your activity, try to eat a balanced meal that includes healthy fats, protein, and carbohydrates. This will offer a consistent supply of energy and lessen the need for food while working out.

2. Consume Complex Carbohydrates : For long-lasting energy, choose complex carbs from foods like whole grains, fruits, and vegetables. A diet high in simple sugars should be avoided because it might lead to energy spikes and crashes.

3. Include Protein : To promote muscle growth and repair, include a reasonable amount of protein in your pre-exercise meal. Lean meats, poultry, fish, eggs, dairy products, legumes, and nuts are all excellent sources of protein.

4. Remain Hydrated : To make sure you're adequately hydrated prior to your workout, drink a lot of water. For most workouts, water is the best option, but if you're working out hard or for a long time, you might want to try a sports drink to replace electrolytes.

5. Limit Fat and Fiber: Steer clear of foods heavy in fat and fiber during exercise since they can slow down digestion and produce discomfort in the stomach. Instead, pick light, easily digested foods that won't burden you.

6. Timing Is Important: Give yourself two to three hours to digest your pre-exercise food before working out. If you have to work out early in the morning or don't have time for a large breakfast, choose to eat a little snack half an hour or so beforehand.

7. Select Well-Digested Foods: Prior to exercising, limit your intake of foods that you know your body can handle. Don't attempt new or strange foods that can make you sick to your stomach.

8. Take into Account the Workout's Intensity and Duration: Your pre-exercise nutritional requirements may be impacted by the workout's intensity and duration. A smaller snack might be plenty for shorter, less strenuous workouts. A larger, more balanced supper could be required after longer or more strenuous exercise.

9. Pay Attention to Your Body: Since every person has a different set of nutritional requirements, it's critical to pay attention to your body and modify your pre-exercise diet accordingly. If you discover that some foods or times are more effective for you, stay with those.

You may maximize your performance and fuel your workouts efficiently by adhering to these pre-exercise nutrition guidelines. Try a variety of foods and times to see what suits you and your fitness objectives the best.

11.3 - POST-WORKOUT DIETARY ADVICE

Nutrition after exercise is essential for promoting recovery and refueling the body with energy. Here are some dietary suggestions for after exercise to help you properly replenish and recuperate:

1. Timing is Crucial : Try to have a protein- and carbohydrate-rich meal or snack 30 to 60 minutes after doing out. This time frame is crucial for refueling glycogen reserves and encouraging muscle development and repair.

2. Replace Fluids : Hydration is essential to replenish fluids lost through perspiration after physical activity. If you want to rehydrate and replace electrolytes, consume water or a sports drink.

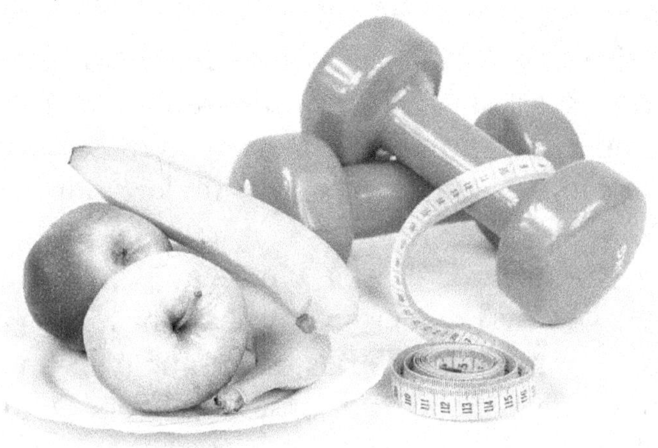

3. Incorporate Protein : Both muscle growth and repair depend on protein. Your post-workout meal or snack should contain a source of protein, such as dairy products, lentils, fish, poultry, eggs, and lean meats or protein drinks.

4. Select carbs Carefully : To restore glycogen stores and offer a consistent supply of energy, choose complex carbs such those found in whole grains, fruits, and vegetables. A diet high in simple sugars should be avoided because it might lead to energy spikes and crashes.

5. Incorporate Healthy Fats: Adding healthy fats to your post-workout meal might help you feel fuller and supply vital nutrients. Pick healthy sources like olive oil, almonds, seeds, and avocados.

6. Take Into Account Your Protein Requirements : Your post-workout protein requirements are influenced by a number of variables, including your body weight, level of exertion, and fitness objectives. Try to have 15–25 grams of protein at each meal or snack.

7. Refuel Electrolytes: If you perspired a lot throughout your workout, you might want to drink a sports drink or eat foods high in electrolytes, such bananas, oranges, and coconut water.

8. Be Mindful of Your Intuition for Hunger and Fullness : After working out, pay attention to your body's signals of hunger and fullness. Eat till you're pleased but not full enough to cause discomfort or hinder your healing process.

9. Recovery Smoothie : For a quick and simple post-workout meal, try a recovery smoothie that is high in protein, carbohydrates, and liquids. Combine everything in a blender, including yogurt, fruit, protein powder inclusive.

10. Whole foods vs. pills : Your main source of post-exercise nourishment should be whole foods, even though pills can be handy. Try not to rely only on supplements to meet your nutrient needs; instead, try eating a balanced diet.

These post-workout meal suggestions can help you recover from your workouts, refuel your energy reserves, and encourage muscle growth and repair. Try a variety of foods and times to see what suits you and your fitness objectives the best.

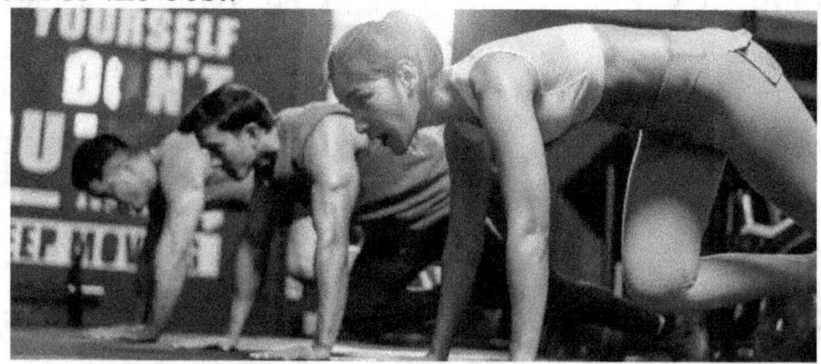

11.4 - GUIDELINES FOR HYDRATION IN PHYSICALLY ACTIVE PEOPLE

Everyone needs to drink enough water, but energetic people who work out frequently really need to do so. Maintaining proper hydration helps avoid dehydration, control body temperature, and sustain peak performance. For those who are active, consider the following hydration guidelines:

1. Drink Water Throughout the Day : It's crucial to stay hydrated all day long, not just when working out. Try to drink 8 to 10 cups (64 to 80 ounces) of water a day, or more if you're moving vigorously or it's really hot outside.

2. Pre-Exercise Hydration : To make sure you're well-hydrated before you begin, drink 17–20 ounces of water two to three hours beforehand. Eight more ounces of water should be had for 20 to 30 minutes before going out.

3. Hydration During Exercise : If you're exercising for more than an hour or in hot conditions, try to drink 7 to 10 ounces of water every 10 to 20 minutes. If you're working out hard or for a long time, think about getting a sports drink to replace the electrolytes you lose through perspiration.

4. Post-activity Hydration : For each pound of body weight lost during activity, consume 16–24 ounces of water. This will assist in replenishing lost fluids from perspiration and rehydrating your body.

5. Check Your Hydration Level : Be alert for symptoms of dehydration, such as headaches, dark urine, dry mouth, or exhaustion. If you feel like you're dehydrated, try drinking more water and taking some time to relax.

6. Take Electrolyte Intake Into Consideration : In addition to drinking water, take into account ingesting foods or beverages that are high in electrolytes, such as coconut water, sports drinks, or electrolyte pills. This can support electrolyte balance maintenance, particularly after extended or vigorous activity.

7. Take into Account the Environment : Sweating during hot and muggy weather can increase fluid loss, thus it's crucial to drink more water during these times. Observe your body's feelings and modify your fluid intake as necessary.

8. Individual Hydration Needs: Individual hydration requirements differ depending on age, gender, weight, fitness level, and surroundings. Pay attention to your body's needs and modify your fluid intake accordingly.

You can perform at your best and maintain your health by adhering to these hydration rules and making sure you're adequately hydrated before, during, and after exercise.

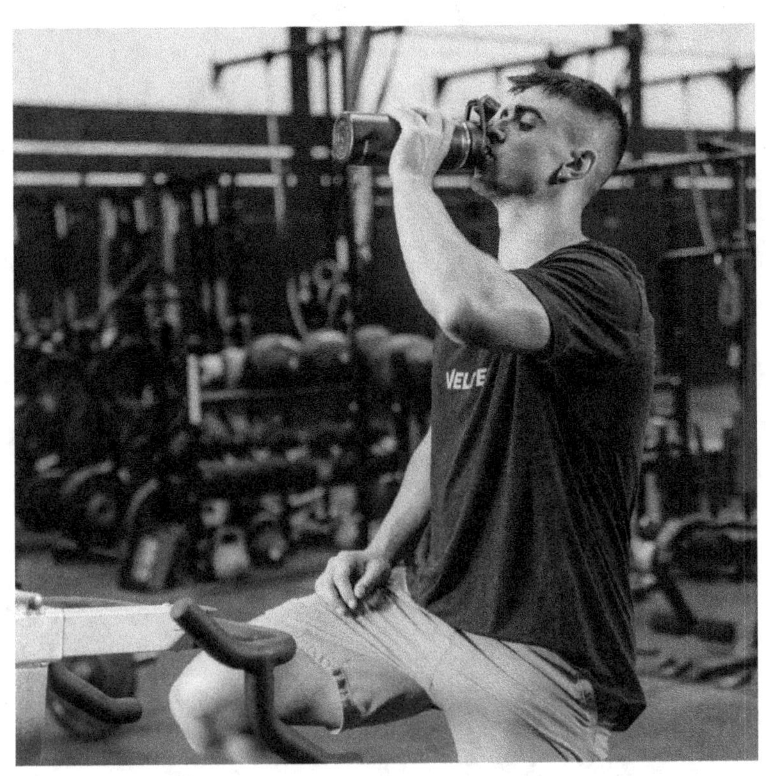

12.0 MIND-BODY CONNECTION IN FITNESS

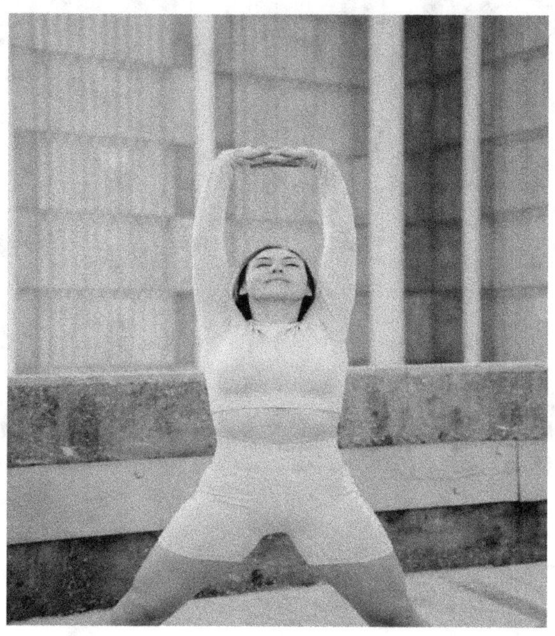

12.1 - IMPORTANCE OF THE MIND-BODY CONNECTION IN FITNESS

Fitness has a strong and sometimes disregarded mind-body connection, which contributes to general wellbeing. It deals with how your body, mind, and emotions interact when you exercise, and it can have a big impact on your fitness goals. You can get better outcomes, feel better mentally, and boost your exercises by realizing and utilizing this link.

The mind-body connection's impact on motivation and consistency in your exercise regimen is one of its main features. You are more likely to maintain your motivation and dedication to your workouts when you are mentally alert and attentive while exercising. You may overcome obstacles and plateaus with the support of this mental focus, improving your performance eventually.

Additionally, the mind-body link can improve your exercise-related physical performance. Research has demonstrated that mental engagement and focus can enhance physical performance. This is due to the fact that your mind can assist you in realizing the full potential of your body, enabling you to work out harder and accomplish more.

Stress and anxiety can also be lessened by the mind-body link. Exercise is well known for its ability to reduce stress, and its effects can be amplified if you approach your workouts with mental awareness. You can relax and feel less stressed and anxious by paying attention to your body's sensations and the pattern of your breathing.

The mind-body link also has the potential to enhance general wellbeing. You can get more enjoyment and fulfillment from your workouts when you are in tune with your body and mind while exercising. This may result in increased self-assurance and a happier perspective on life.

It is crucial to practice mindfulness and present during your workouts in order to develop a strong mind-body connection in your fitness program. This entails paying attention to your body's feelings, such as how your muscles feel and how your breath rhythms. It also entails observing your feelings and ideas objectively and letting them come and go without being attached to them.

Including exercises like tai chi, yoga, or meditation can also improve the mind-body connection. Through these exercises, you can develop a deeper connection with your body and mind and learn to be more mindful of the present moment. Finding fun and fulfilling hobbies can also improve your mind-body connection and increase the enjoyment of your workouts.

To sum up, the mind-body link is an effective tool that can improve your general health and fitness experience. You may reach your body's maximum potential, lessen tension and anxiety, and get more enjoyment and fulfillment out of your workouts by practicing mindfulness and present.

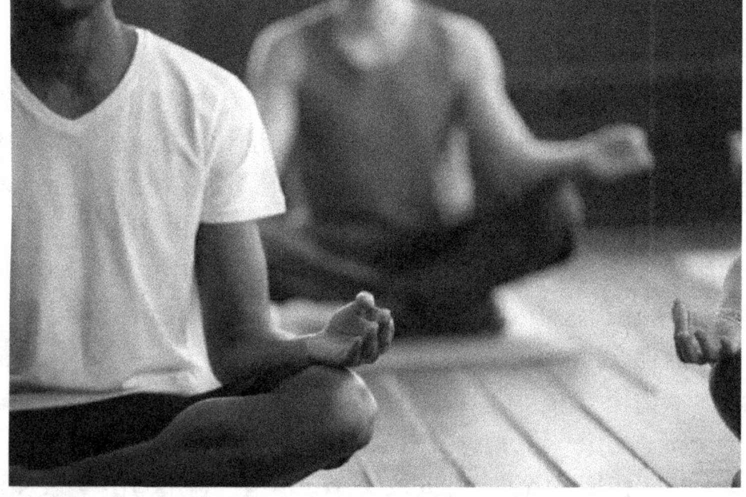

12.2 - ADVANTAGES OF YOGA AND MEDITATION TECHNIQUES

Numerous health benefits are provided for the body and mind by engaging in practices like yoga and meditation. Stress reduction is one of the main advantages of these techniques. The mind-calming, anxiety-reduction, and cortisol-lowering effects of yoga and meditation have been linked to improved general health and wellbeing.

Yoga and meditation can also help with strength, balance, and flexibility. Stretches and postures used in yoga, in particular, help increase the flexibility and mobility of the muscles and joints. On the other hand, focus and concentration can be enhanced through meditation, which can be advantageous for cognitive function and general mental clarity.

Additionally, yoga and meditation might enhance the quality of your sleep. These practices incorporate relaxation techniques that can assist soothe the body and mind, which can facilitate falling asleep and staying asleep all night. This may result in more restorative sleep and higher overall sleep quality.

Moreover, attention and self-awareness are enhanced by yoga and meditation. By using these techniques, you can develop a stronger sense of self-awareness and learn to live in the present. This can raise your sense of general well-being and make you feel more confident and good about yourself.

Lastly, practicing yoga and meditation can help with chronic pain management. Research has indicated that these techniques can assist in lowering pain levels and enhancing quality of life for those with ailments such as back ache, fibromyalgia and arthritis.

In the end, physical and mental health can benefit greatly from disciplines like yoga and meditation. These exercises can benefit general health and wellbeing by reducing stress and promoting flexibility and balance. Including yoga and meditation in your daily practice can improve your life, relaxation, and attention both on and off the mat.

12.3 - THE RELATIONSHIP BETWEEN MENTAL AND PHYSICAL HEALTH

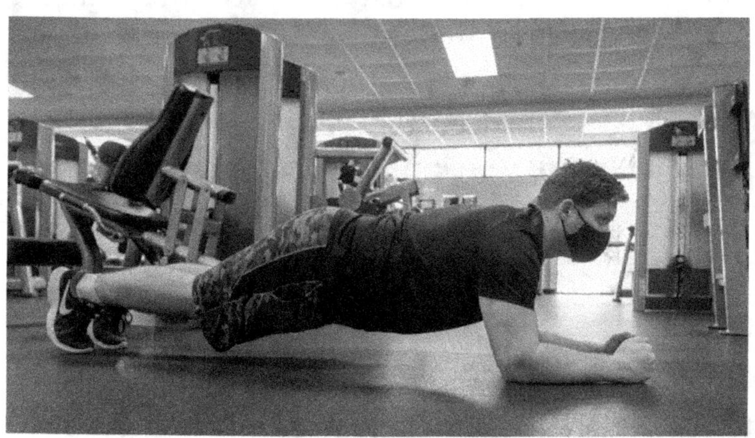

There is a complicated and reciprocal relationship between physical and mental health. Both physical and mental health can have a significant influence on one another. The following are some ways that physical and mental health are correlated:

1. The relationship between mental and physical health : - A variety of physical health issues can be attributed to mental health disorders such stress, anxiety, and depression.

- For instance, long-term stress can raise inflammation in the body, which is connected to diseases including diabetes, autoimmune disorders, and heart disease.

- Because they impair immunity and increase a person's susceptibility to infections and illnesses, depression and anxiety can also have an impact on one's physical health.

- Furthermore, lifestyle choices like food, exercise, and sleep are significant factors that determine one's physical health and can be impacted by mental health conditions.

2. Effect of Physical Health on Mental Health: Issues with one's physical well-being can also have a big effect on one's mental well-being.

Feelings of irritation, loneliness, and helplessness can result from long-term illnesses or disabilities.

Anxiety brought on by physical health difficulties might also exacerbate mental health problems.

- Moreover, occasionally the adverse effects of drugs taken to address physical illnesses can make mental health issues worse.

3. Biological principles : The connection between physical and mental health is based on biological principles.

- Stress, for instance, triggers the hypothalamic-pituitary-adrenal (HPA) axis, which releases stress hormones like cortisol. These chemicals can affect the body in a number of ways, including elevated blood pressure and weakened immune system performance. Chronic activation of the stress response system may eventually have a role in the emergence of physical health issues.

4. Behavioral Factors : - The connection between physical and mental health is also influenced by behavioral factors.

- For instance, people with mental health difficulties may be more prone to harmful habits like smoking, eating poorly, and not exercising, all of which can exacerbate physical health issues. On the other hand, regular physical activity can improve mental health by lowering anxiety and depressive symptoms.

In summary, there is a close relationship between mental and physical health, and each can have a big influence on the other. Prioritizing your physical and emotional well-being is crucial, and you should get help from medical specialists when you need it to deal with any potential problems.

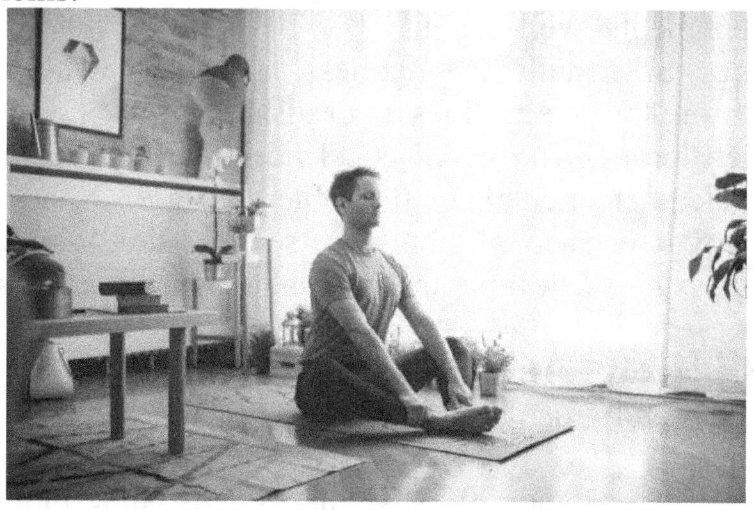

12.4 - TECHNIQUES FOR ENHANCING THE PHYSICAL-MENTAL BOND THROUGH EXERCISE

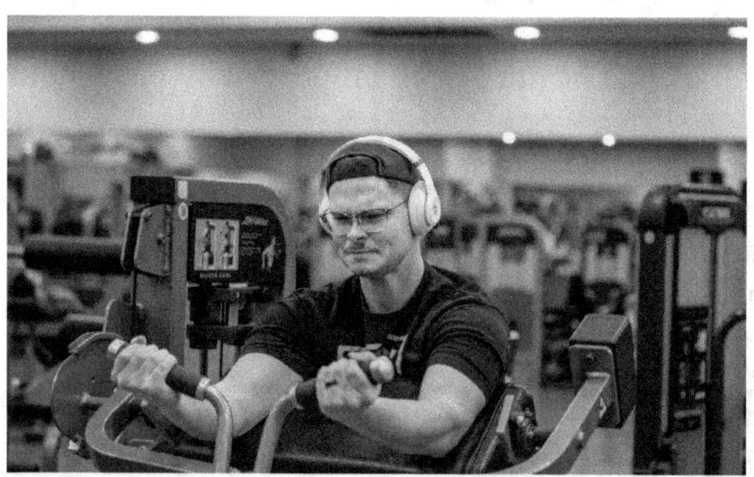

Developing awareness and presence while exercising is a key component of strengthening the mind-body connection. The following are some methods to strengthen this bond:

1. Keep Your Mind in the Present: When exercising, pay attention to your body's feelings rather than allowing your thoughts to stray. Observe your body's movement, the sensation of your muscles, and the cadence of your breathing.

2. Incorporate Mindful Movement: Take part in activities like yoga, tai chi, or qigong that encourage mindfulness. These exercises focus on slow, intentional movements that support body-mind awareness.

3. Employ Breath Awareness : Throughout your workout, be mindful of your breathing. To help you relax and bring your attention to the here and now, practice diaphragmatic breathing.

4. Body Cues Mindfulness : During physical activity, pay attention to your body's cues by listening to it. If something hurts or seems awkward, change how you're moving or, if needed, stop and rest.

5. Involve Your Senses : When exercising, use your senses to establish a connection with your surroundings. To improve your sensory experience, pay attention to the sights, sounds, and fragrances around you.

6. Set Intentions: Make a plan for your exercise session before you begin. This could be an emphasis on self-improvement, thankfulness, or just being in the present.

7. Engage in Visualization Practice : Envision yourself executing exercises with elegance and ease. This can strengthen your mind-body connection and help you with form and technique.

8. Combine workout with Mindfulness Practices: To improve the mind-body connection, incorporate mindfulness exercises like meditation or deep breathing into your workout regimen.

9. Examine Your Experience : After working out, pause to consider your bodily and emotional well-being. This can increase your awareness of the relationship between your body and mind.

10. Have patience and perseverance : It takes practice and time to establish a strong mind-body connection. Have patience with yourself and keep using these techniques on a regular basis in your workout regimen.

You can improve the physical and mental effects of your workouts and strengthen the mind-body connection by implementing these techniques into your regimen.